T0136098

Bulimia
Nervosa

JAMES E. MITCHELL, M.D.

University of Minnesota Press
Minneapolis

Published by the University of Minnesota Press
2037 University Avenue Southeast, Minneapolis, MN 55414
Printed in the United States of America

Library of Congress Cataloging-in-Publication Data

Mitchell, James E. (James Edward), 1947–
    Bulimia nervosa / James E. Mitchell.
        p.   cm.
    Summary: Bibliography: p.
    Includes index.
    ISBN 0-8166-1626-4
    1. Bulimia.   I. Title.
    [DNLM: 1. Bulimia—therapy.   WM 175 M681b]
    RC552.B84M57 1989
    616.85'263 – dc20
    DNLM/DLC   89-5057
for Library of Congress   CIP

The University of Minnesota
is an equal-opportunity
educator and employer.

To my wife, Karen,

and

To Burtrum Shiele, M.D., my first teacher in psychiatry,
who introduced me to psychiatric research and
who always demonstrated a respect for the necessity of
integrity in science and a genuine concern
for both his patients and his students.

Contents

Preface

Why another book on eating disorders? A fair question, given the veritable cornucopia of works in this area, some of high quality, and others more marginal, published over the last decade. I decided to write this book for several reasons. First, there have been few books devoted exclusively to bulimia nervosa. Most of the published work focuses on anorexia nervosa. The relative paucity of books on bulimia nervosa reflects the fact that we have been studying this disorder for a much shorter period of time than anorexia nervosa, despite the fact that bulimia nervosa is a more prevalent condition. Second, I wished to write a book that experienced clinicians could read carefully and afterwards feel that they had a clear sense of the disorder and a general understanding as to how to treat it. Therefore, this work is practical rather than theoretical, and is written primarily for practitioners, be they physicians who wish to become familiar with the disorder and its medical complications, psychiatrists who wish to do psychotherapy with or administer pharmacotherapy to these patients, psychologists or social workers who work with these patients in the clinic or in the hospital, or other health professionals or educators who wish an overview of the disorder.

My third reason for writing this book was to force myself to review much of the literature on this disorder, and to attempt to synthesize it in a way that would be understandable to me and, I hope to others as well. Those of us who devote a good portion of our time to research frequently find ourselves becoming highly expert in obscure areas and poorly informed on important, related topics. Therefore, much of this writing was done in the service of my own knowledge and updating.

The book focuses on the assessment and treatment of adult women with bulimia nervosa who are of approximately normal weight and who are mature and independent enough to be treated in individual or group therapy rather than family therapy. Therefore, there are many areas that are not addressed or are addressed only superficially. Very little discussion is devoted to the treatment of bulimia nervosa in individuals who also meet criteria for anorexia nervosa, or individuals with obesity who have bulimic symptoms. Bulimia nervosa is rare in males, and only a limited space is devoted to that topic. Also the text focuses on the treatment of adults. Those who work primarily with adolescents or with families will need additional information from other sources. Because the largest subgroup of individuals who seek treatment for this disorder are adult, normal-weight women, I will use the female pronoun throughout the text.

Certain theoretical biases underlying this work will soon become obvious to most readers. The point of view is descriptive rather than psychodynamic. While I am more than willing to acknowledge that psychodynamic formulations may explain or help to explain the psychopathology of many individuals with bulimia nervosa, it seems to me that dynamic models are not yet well enough developed to allow for practical clinical application for this condition in most settings. I think that a descriptive, behavioral model currently provides the most useful means to understand, manage, and treat these patients. I also believe that pharmacotherapy is a very useful adjunct in the treatment of many of these patients. Lastly, I believe that those who care for these patients must be closely attuned to the fact that many of them are medically ill and need medical monitoring and supervision. This is a role that many non-M.D. therapists find uncomfortable. Nonetheless, all therapists who are involved in the care of these patients need to ensure that such monitoring is accomplished.

Our understanding of bulimia nervosa has grown dramatically since 1979, when Gerald Russell first delineated the problem. Much has been learned, but many important, even crucial questions remain. As I wrote this book, I was somewhat saddened by the knowledge that as soon as it could be published it would be out of date. Things are moving quickly in this area, and I urge readers who read this book and wish to have the latest information on this disorder to supplement their reading by carefully perusing the most recent journal references on the topic.

A thread that I have attempted to weave throughout this book and have communicated repeatedly is the need for an understanding and compassionate stance with these patients. I remember the first time I interviewed a woman with bulimia nervosa. It was 1978, and I was in private psychiatric practice, fresh from my residency. A woman I was seeing for depression confessed to me that she was actively bulimic. I had never heard of the problem, was taken aback by what she described, and offered her the advice that I am sure many therapists before and since have also offered such patients: "Why don't you just quit?" Most of these individuals cannot just quit. They have a behavioral disorder that requires compassion, understanding, support, encouragement, and therapy. Given these elements, most can "quit." I hope that this book will promulgate practical observations and techniques that will be of use to the therapists who treat these patients.

Minneapolis   James E. Mitchell, M.D.

Acknowledgments

To acknowledge and thank one's colleagues in a medical text such as this is quite different from acknowledgments made in the preface of a novel. A novelist may receive considerable help from others in constructing his or her manuscript, but the ideas are basically the writer's own. That is not true in science. Most everything in this text was thought of and written about by others, and much of it is probably explained better elsewhere. All I have done is attempt to prioritize the material, at times to make critical judgments about the importance of the studies involved, and to synthesize it all in a way that will be palatable to readers. By extension, it would be facetious for me to try to thank everyone who contributed to this book.

Instead I will acknowledge and thank those with whom I have worked and those whose work I have most admired. First, I would like to thank the other members of the eating disorders research group at the University of Minnesota, including Richard L. Pyle, M.D., Elke D. Eckert, M.D., Dorothy Hatsukami, Ph.D., and Claire Pomeroy, M.D. Each contributed substantially to the treatment recommendations outlined in this book. One could not ask for more creative, supportive colleagues, and I have enjoyed our collaborations immensely. Second, I would like to thank Paula Clayton, M.D., the chair of my department, who has been unfailingly supportive and helpful with her advice during my tenure at the University of Minnesota. Third, I would like to thank the therapists who have worked with our program and have been responsible for conducting much of the psychotherapy research that our group has produced. In particular, I would like to thank Gretchen Goff, M.A., Jane Harper, M.S.W., Debbie Glotter, M.S.W., and Mary Zollman, R.D., all of whom have worked with the program for several years and have made significant contributions to the therapy manuals developed at Minnesota. Lana Boutacoff, M.A., a former therapist with our program, was particularly instrumental in manual development, and our entire group owes her a large debt of gratitude. I would also like to thank the research assistants who have worked with our group over the last seven years. In particular I would like to mention Kelli Skoog, research coordinator; Marguerite Huber, nurse practitioner; Elizabeth Soll; Linda Fletcher; and Kyle Lundby, each of whom has had a very important role in my research efforts. Fourth, I would like to thank Kris Ullereng and Janet Bockenstedt, who typed the manuscripts, answered the phones, and managed the office. I have never had better secretarial support. Last, I would like to thank several of my professional colleagues. A subgroup of these individuals have been particularly important to me; each has given to me freely of ideas and time and has strongly influenced my work. I had anticipated that life in academics would be fiercely competitive. Instead, I have encountered friendliness and openness. These people include Kelly Bemis, Ph.D., University of Hawaii; Christopher Fairburn, M.D., Oxford University; Manfred Fichter, M.D., University of Munich; David Garner, Ph.D., Michigan State University; David Hertzog, M.D., Massachusetts General Hospital, Harvard University; Katherine Halmi, M.D., Cornell University; Craig Johnson, M.D., Northwestern University; Walter Kaye, M.D., University of Pittsburgh and Western Psychiatric Institute; David Jimerson, M.D., Beth Israel Hospital Harvard University; and B. Timothy Walsh, M.D., Columbia University.

There are several other individuals whom I have known less well, but who are leaders in this field and who have been helpful to me, both directly and through their work. These include include Stuart Agras, M.D., Stanford University; Arnold Anderson, M.D., Johns Hopkins University; Peter Beumont, M.D., University of Sydney,; Regina Casper, M.D., University of Chicago; Paul Garfinkel, M.D., University of Toronto; Laurie Humphries, M.D., University of Kentucky; Gloria Leon, Ph.D., University of Minnesota; James Hudson, M.D. and Harrison Pope, M.D., Maclean Hospital, Belmont, Mass., and Harvard Medical School; Karl Pirke, M.D., Max Planck Institute, Munich; Michael Strober, Ph.D. and Joel Yaeger, M.D., University of California, Los Angeles; Walter Vandereycken, M.D., Kortenberg, Belgium; and Terry Wilson, Ph.D., Rutgers University, New Brunswick, N.J.

Bulimia Nervosa

1

An Overview of Bulimia Nervosa

Our initial task is to define bulimia nervosa. However, before we can meaningfully discuss criteria for this disorder, we need to first decide on a frame of reference. What type of model best describes this disorder? Should bulimia nervosa be regarded as a disease? This construct, which presupposes some underlying pathophysiology and a predictable course, is the model used in the current view of schizophrenia and primary affective disorder and in most of medicine. Unfortunately this model does not fit well with much of what is known about bulimia nervosa. No one has yet been able to delineate a specific pathophysiology for this condition, or a specific, predictable, longitudinal course.

Perhaps bulimia nervosa is best viewed as a variant of some other illness? Two models, related to this position, have been put forth, and will be discussed in more detail later. One is that bulimia nervosa is actually a variant of affective disorder;[156,184] the alternative model is that it is a variant of alcohol/drug (substance) abuse.[38] Certainly there is evidence that a high percentage of patients with bulimia nervosa are depressed,[156] and that drug abuse problems are quite common among these individuals compared to the rate of such problems in the general population.[300] However, neither of these models appear to fully explain bulimia nervosa, although research guided by these models has and will continue to contribute to our understanding of the subgroups of the disorder.

Perhaps bulimia nervosa should be regarded as a manifestation of some biological abnormality? Perhaps, but still to be proven. A cultural phenomena? To some extent. There is evidence that the disorder is culturally linked,[31] but all young females in the cultures where bulimia nervosa

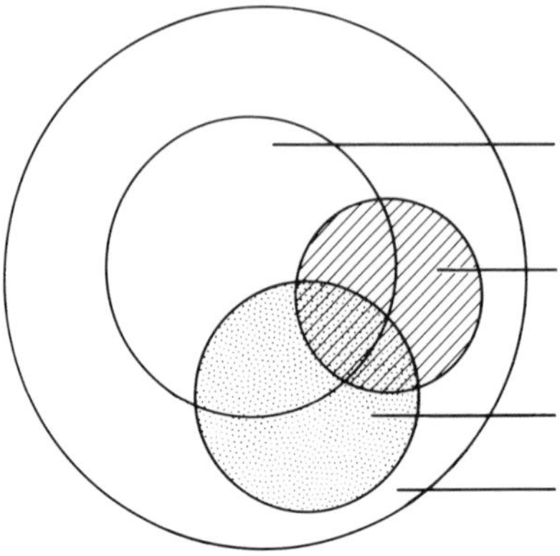

Figure 1. Cormorbidity in Individuals with Bulimia Nervosa

is common do not develop bulimia nervosa. A manifestation of a personality disorder? There is evidence that some bulimic patients have personality disorders,[214] but certainly not all of them.

If we reject these other formulations as unsatisfactory explanations, we are left with the construct that bulimia nervosa, as we now can understand it, probably should be viewed simply as a behavioral disorder — a grouping of problem behaviors — and it seems to me that this is where the current literature leads us. We know that patients with bulimia nervosa, as currently defined, demonstrate certain behaviors in various combinations and at various frequencies, and that the practice of these behaviors, over time, is associated with the development of certain predictable psychosocial sequelae, including low self-esteem and depression. However, in working with patients who have this disorder, one quickly observes that although the behaviors may be similar, in other ways this is a very heterogeneous group of patients. Some are not depressed, and some maintain adequate self-esteem; the differences among patients are as striking as the similarities. It would be comforting if we had a simple, explanatory model for this disorder, but for now, it seems to me that we are stuck with a purely descriptive model.

My own current view, which I will be happy to amend as our knowledge improves, is that bulimia nervosa is a behavioral disorder that can occur as a complicating feature in other disorders, as a symptom in association with certain personality disorders, or as a problem in individuals who do not have other psychological or behavioral problems but who develop bulimic behaviors because of cultural factors. I also think that bulimia nervosa varies as to severity and duration, and has a highly vari-able outcome. I have summarized some of these overlaping constructs in-volving associated psychopathology in figure 1. I'm not at all sure of the relative size of the circles, or the degree of overlap, and I am sure other circles will eventually be added to this model.

Of utmost importance to our understanding of this disorder is the fact that there are two variables that are highly correlated with its develop-ment. The cultural variable—this disorder occurs almost exclusively in societies in which there is a high emphasis placed on thinness[33,34,402]— and gender—this disorder occurs almost exclusively in women.[83,143, 213,422]

Cultural Variables

The importance of cultural variables is difficult to prove, but several lines of evidence suggest this association. First is the growing evidence that bulimia nervosa has become more common and that this increase appears to be confined to industrialized societies that have an excess of food.[334,213] Second, there is much evidence to suggest that there is a cultural preoccu-pation with thinness in many of these same societies. During much of recorded history weight signified security and wealth, but this model is no longer valid in many western societies. Now slimness, which is seen as synonymous with self-discipline and control, is the desired goal.[428] This has happened despite the fact that, on average people weigh more than they did two or three decades ago, and we are left with a growing disparity between actual body weight and desired weight particularly for young women. The increasing emphasis on thinness as a model of attractiveness is also suggested by other observable phenomena in our society, such as the portrayal of women in art and advertising. Third, this growing preoc-cupation with slimness has caused girls and young women to feel over-weight or fat, even if they are of normal weight, which has led to a high percentage of young women who develop abnormal eating-related be-haviors, as will be reviewed in the section on epidemiology. Fourth, what little cross-cultural work is available suggests that in societies where there is less of an emphasis on thinness, these disorders are very rare indeed.

Johnson and Maddi[213] have discussed other cultural variables that may be involved. Women now at risk for eating disorders are really the first generation of women to grow up during a time of dramatic changes in so-ciety's perceptions of women's roles. These young women are expected

Table 1. Russell's Diagnostic Criteria for Bulimia Nervosa

A. Bulimia nervosa – Original Criteria[390]
 1. The patients suffer from powerful and intractable urges to overeat.
 2. They seek to avoid the "fattening" effects of food by inducing vomiting or abusing purgatives or both.
 3. They have a morbid fear of becoming fat.
B. Bulimia Nervosa – Russell's Revised Criteria[105]
 1. Preoccupation with food, irresistible cravings for food and repeated episodes of overeating.
 2. Devices aimed at counteracting the "fattening" effects of food.
 3. A psychopathology resembling that of classical anorexia nervosa.
 4. A previous overt or cryptic episode of anorexia nervosa.

to be attractive and domestic in traditional feminine roles, yet also to be independent and to seek vocational parity with men. Although difficult to prove, it seems quite plausible that such expectations have led to identity confusion and may have contributed to the development of these disorders.

Diagnosis

The diagnostic systems for bulimia nervosa are still in the process of evolution, in part owing to a lack of knowledge about this disorder.[148] The concept of bulimia nervosa as a separate, distinct problem was first elaborated in 1979 by Russell, who emphasized the relationship between this disorder and anorexia nervosa.[390] His original criteria strongly emphasized concerns about shape and weight, also concerns for those with anorexia nervosa (table 1). Also, binge-eating was not originally required for the diagnosis, although these criteria were subsequently revised for both clinical and research purposes to include binge-eating (table 2).[391]

Bulimia was first recognized as a separate disorder in the American Psychiatric Association nomenclature in the 1980 DSM-III. The original criteria, summarized in table 2, reflected an emphasis on binge-eating behavior; associated features such as vomiting and laxative abuse were not required for the diagnosis, and there was no criterion concerning preoccupation with shape and weight. The Russell criteria and the American Psy-

Table 2. Diagnostic Criteria for DSM-III Bulimia

A. Recurrent episodes of binge-eating (rapid consumption of a large amount of food in a discrete period of time, usually less than two hours).

B. At least three of the following:

  1. consumption of high-caloric, easily ingested food during a binge
  2. inconspicuous eating during a binge
  3. termination of such eating episodes by abdominal pain, sleep, social interruption, or self-induced vomiting
  4. repeated attempts to lose weight by severely restrictive diets, self-induced vomiting, or use of cathartics or diuretics
  5. frequent weight fluctuations greater than 10 pounds due to alternating binges and fasts.

C. Awareness that the eating pattern is abnormal and fear of not being able to stop eating voluntarily.

D. Depressed mood and self-deprecating thoughts following eating binges.

E. Bulimic episodes not due to anorexia nervosa or any known physical disorder.

Table 3. Diagnostic Criteria for DSM-III-R Bulimia Nervosa

A. Recurrent episodes of binge-eating (rapid consumption of a large amount of food in a discrete period of time).

B. A feeling of lack of control over eating behavior during the eating binges.

C. The person regularly engages in either self-induced vomiting, use of laxatives or diuretics, strict dieting or fasting, or vigorous exercise in order to prevent weight gain.

D. A minimum average of two binge-eating episodes a week for at least three months.

E. Persistent overconcern with body shape and weight.

chiatric Association criteria have come closer in the DSM-III-R, summarized in table 3.[82] As can be seen, binge-eating is still required for the diagnosis, although the construct of binge-eating remains somewhat vague. Unfortunately, disagreement exists as to how to define an eating binge, although guidelines have been suggested by Fairburn.[99, 105]

This lack of agreement is one major problem in clinical work and research on this disorder. One criterion in DSM-III-R, requires some behavior, either active (such as vomiting or laxative abuse) or passive (such as fasting), designed to counteract the effects of the eating binge. However, series of patients with bulimia nervosa are composed almost exclu-

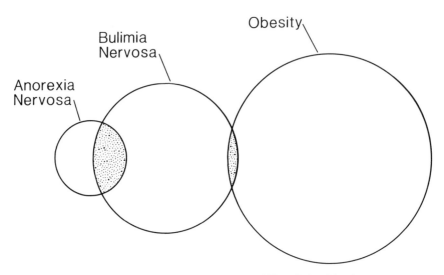

Figure 2. Overlap and Relative Prevalence of Three Eating Disorders

sively of individuals whose binge-eating is coupled with self-induced vomiting or laxative abuse, and vomiting or laxative abuse are prerequisites for participation in many research studies. Individuals who engage exclusively in the other types of behaviors, such as exercising and fasting, are seen less commonly in eating disorder clinics, and we really know little about these other subgroups and how they relate to patients who vomit or use laxatives.

Let us now turn to the relationship between bulimia nervosa and other clinical eating disorders. In figure 2 I have diagrammed the relationships among anorexia nervosa, bulimia nervosa, and obesity, the size of the circles roughly suggesting the relative prevalence of the disorders. The circles from left to right indicate relative weight, with individuals who have anorexia nervosa being underweight, most patients with bulimia nervosa being of normal weight, and patients with obesity being overweight. As can be seen, there is considerable overlap. The overlap between anorexia nervosa and bulimia nervosa is dealt with differently in the DSM-III-R than it was in the DSM-III.[82] Individuals who meet criteria for both disorders are now assigned both diagnoses, whereas in DSM-III the diagnosis of anorexia nervosa took precedence. Patients who have anorexia nervosa yet also have bulimic symptoms in many ways resemble normal-weight bulimics more than underweight restrictor anorectics.[120,123,124,126]

As suggested by figure 2, there is also overlap between bulimia nervosa and obesity, and the boundaries can vary depending on the criteria employed.[372] This subgroup has been studied very little,[191,236,286] and the differences between this group and normal-weight bulimic patients have yet to be adequately elucidated. However, it is known that overweight bulimics appear to have the same risk for affective disorder as normal-weight bulimics, but are less likely to use vomiting as a weight-control technique.[191]

Many eating problems that occur in normal-weight individuals are not classified as eating disorders in the DSM-III-R. This classification system makes it possible to define and discuss syndromes that are, to some extent, fairly behaviorally homogeneous, but the system omits some important eating problems. For example, what is compulsive overeating? What about individuals who exercise excessively and are overly rigid about their eating behavior, but never engage in binging or purging, and never lose a large amount of weight? What about people who believe themselves to have allergies to food and who have peculiar eating patterns and food choices, yet never satisfy criteria for bulimia nervosa or anorexia nervosa? What about those who self-induce vomiting or use laxatives or diuretics for weight control purposes but never binge-eat, or have binge-eaten in the past but have ceased the behavior? Clearly there are many other subgroups that are not adequately addressed by the current criteria. Frankly we know little about most of the groups, other than that they can seriously challenge the resourcefulness of therapists. However, we will try to discuss several of these problems later in the sections on treatment.

Demography

The descriptions of several series of women with bulimia nervosa have been published in the literature, and from these reports we can extract a composite picture of the disorder. The descriptive information from four surveys that included at least 100 subjects is summarized in table 4.[102,216,300,313] In examining these data, certain themes become apparent. First, bulimia nervosa is much more common among women than men. This holds true across bulimia treatment centers and, although cross-cultural data are quite limited now, across countries. Second, the typical age of onset clusters around 18, although the disorder can begin much earlier.[162,163] The mean onset age of 18 is fairly consistent across studies and suggests that this disorder is precipitated at the time when young

Table 4. Characteristics of Reported Series of Bulimic Individuals

Authors	Sex		Age X		Binge-eat		Vomit	
	Male	Female	At study	At onset	Daily->	Weekly->	Daily->	Weekly->
Fairburn & Cooper 1982 (N=499)	0%	100%	23.8	18.4	27.2%	32.6%	56.1%	17.5%
Johnson et al. 1982 (N=316)	0%	100%	23.7	18.1	51.5%	41.8%	59.2%	28.6%
Mitchell et al. 1983 (N=168)	2%	98%	24.0	20.0	63.8%	26.7%	56.6%	23.2%
Mitchell et al. 1985 (N=275)	0%	100%	24.8	17.7	82.0%	16.1%	71.8%	12.2%

*Origin of research subjects: Fairburn & Cooper—responded to advertisement; Johnson—wrote clinic; Mitchell, 1983 & 1985—patients consulted doctors with eating disorder symptoms.

x=mean.

women are leaving home to enter the work force or to begin college. In most series, the majority of patients have never married; but the condition usually puts considerable strain on the relationships of married bulimic patients.[446]

The mean duration of illness before seeking treatment is surprisingly long in most surveys, often six or seven years. The reasons for this have not been adequately studied, but several considerations may be relevant. First, the longer people are actively symptomatic with bulimia nervosa, the worse their eating symptoms become. Also, it has been observed that the longer patients have active bulimia nervosa the more likely they are to gain weight.[96] This weight gain may convince the individual of the futility of her behaviors, which are usually designed to promote weight loss, and therefore serve as a stimulus to seek therapy. It is also reasonable to hypothesize that the longer an individual has bulimia nervosa, the more likely she is to develop secondary psychological and social problems; many seek treatment because of depression, social impairment, or declining academic or work performance rather than for the eating symptoms per se.

Epidemiology

Estimates of the prevalence of this disorder have varied widely. Some reports in the lay press have gone so far as to suggest that the majority of college-age women develop this disorder. This is clearly an exaggeration. The great disparity in prevalence estimates is mainly attributable to variations in definition, and one can obtain widely different figures depending on how vague or how tight the criteria.

To my knowledge, no large population-based survey has examined the prevalence of this disorder in the general population. Most of the studies published to date have involved the administration of questionnaires to selected populations, usually high school or college students. While such studies have been useful in helping to define the magnitude of the problem in the population, they have not told us anything definitive about the true prevalence in the general population, and such a general population study is clearly indicated.

It is useful to examine the available studies in some detail.[53,54,64,68,69,73, 88,136,152,153,158,159,165,169,215,225,232,237,269,280,324,326, 329,364,365,368,369,370,371,373,398,406,418,440,443,450,486,487] Most of the surveys have been of college students, presumably because the college and

Table 5. Prevalence of Binge-Eating, Bulimia, and Bulimia Nervosa in Various Populations

	High School Surveys (4 studies)	College Surveys (18 studies)	Graduate School Surveys (1 study)	Family Practice Clinic (2 studies)	Suburban Shoppers (1 study)	Working Women (1 study)
Total N	3,160	14,713	550	740	300	139
$\bar{x}$ percent female	68	82	100	100	100	100
$\bar{x}$ percent male	32	18	0	0	0	0
$\bar{x}$ percent response	92	72	50	93	99	46
$\bar{x}$ percent binge-eat						
Female	57	62		26		41
Male		52				
$\bar{x}$ percent DSM-III						
Female	7	10			10	
Male	0	<1				
$\bar{x}$ percent DSM-III-R						
Female		2	2			
Male		>1				
$\bar{x}$ percent research criteria						
Female	1	3	10	1		1
Male	0					

medical school faculty who have done most of this work have access to such populations.

The results of 27 of these studies are summarized in table 5. I have presented the data in several tiers, which reflect different ways of defining the problem. The first tier, summarizes the percentages of males and females surveyed in each study and the percentages responding, if responses were contingent on subject cooperation. The next four tiers show the percentages identified as symptomatic based on different conceptualizations of bulimia or bulimia nervosa. First, does the subject admit to binge-eating? This term has been defined in various ways in different questionnaires, and it is difficult to tell how patients interpret questions about binge-eating. However, in examining these figures, it is clear that a history of binge-eating, when broadly defined, is endorsed by a significant minority or a majority of students. This suggests that endorsement of binge-eating on a questionnaire cannot be used as the sole criterion to identify pathological eating behavior.

In the third tier are data from studies in which an attempt was made to operationalized DSM-III criteria for bulimia, and in the fourth tier DSM-III-R criteria for bulimia nervosa. The last tier reflects studies that have presented data using research criteria, such as requiring the presence of binge-eating coupled with self-induced vomiting or laxative abuse on a regular basis, usually once or twice a week.

As I stated previously, binge-eating is quite common, and DSM-III bulimia, as identified using the criteria employed in these surveys, is certainly common as well, with as many as 20 percent of surveyed females meeting criteria in some studies. However, DSM-III-R bulimia nervosa, and research criteria for bulimia nervosa, are less common, and are probably present in only 1 to 3 percent of surveyed females. They are rare indeed among surveyed men.

To summarize, in considering these studies, self-endorsed binge-eating on questionnaires usually does not indicate a significant eating problem. In attempting to find significant eating problems such as bulimia nervosa, it is more important to include criteria that address frequency, such as two episodes a week as defined in DSM-III-R, and the presence of pathological weight-reduction techniques, such as self-induced vomiting or laxative abuse. These are the symptoms that characterize the eating problems of patients with bulimia nervosa and are most suggestive of the disorder in individuals in the population at large.

Table 6. Bulimia Nervosa Follow-up Studies

Year	Authors	In/Outpatients	Duration	N	Percentage of Success*
1983	Abraham et al.	Out	14–72 months	43	29–42
1983	Lacey	Out	"Up to 2 years"	28	87
1985	Pope et al.	Out	2–28 months	20	50
1985	Swift et al.	In	25–30 months	30	13
1986	Hsu and Holder	Out	12–35 months	48	50
1986	Mitchell et al.	Out	12–15 months	75	
1986	Norman et al.	Out	12 months	37	
1986	Norman and Herzog	Out	24–36 months	18	
1986	Wilson et al.	Out	6 months	10	40
1988	Herzog et al.	Out	6 months	30	33

*Defined differently in individual studies.

Very little information has been published on socioeconomic factors of bulimia nervosa. Based on clinical experience, we can conclude that women from all socioeconomic groups can develop bulimia nervosa.[11,83] However, one study by Pope et al. in 1983 suggested that bulimia nervosa actually may be more common in lower socioeconomic groups.[357]

Longitudinal Course

Very little is known now about the longitudinal course of bulimia nervosa. Investigators have been studying this disorder for a much shorter period than anorexia nervosa, and they have not had enough time to assess long-term outcome and sequelae. The topic has recently been reviewed by Herzog and colleagues, who are now engaged in a large, long-term follow-up study.[166] The available follow-up studies reported in the literature are summarized in table 6.[4,168,179,252,297,335,337,361,433,434] It is important to remember that the duration to follow-up, methodology, and criteria for improvement varied markedly among these reports. Also, the treatments that were administered at baseline also varied, and in some of the series many patients were not treated, but simply evaluated. As summarized in the table, the results suggest that this is a disorder that many times does not remit spontaneously, even over several years' time. However, as documented by Yager and colleagues, some individuals do recover without treatment.[484] As we will see in the chapters on treatment, recent re-

search using certain specific techniques suggest a more favorable outcome, although again the database at this point is still quite limited.

A study of relapse in our 12- to 15-month study suggested that most patients who relapse following treatment do so in the first few months, and
almost all who will relapse have done so by 6 months.[296]

2

Bulimic Behavior

Let us address the core behavioral symptoms of bulimia nervosa, beginning with the hallmark of the disorder—binge-eating. The binge-eating behavior usually starts during a period of restrictive dieting, when the individual loses control and overeats.[160,356,463] The onset can also be associated with stressful life events.[56]

We have previously mentioned the lack of a precise definition for binge-eating, and that this imprecision results in a major stumbling block to research. It would be convenient if binge-eating clearly differed from "normal" eating or "overeating" (another currently undefinable construct), but on the spectrum of eating, binge-eating must merge with overeating. To make matters worse, what some patients report as binge-eating is, on careful questioning, really only eating a normal meal or even a small amount of food. This lack of specificity has contributed to a number of the problems in the prevalence studies of eating disorders, since questionnaires inquiring about binge-eating tend to use different, often imprecise, definitions, and many investigators have not been able to ensure that they are clearly delineating pathological eating behavior.

Questionnaire studies that have examined the self-reported prevalence of binge-eating in select populations have found that between 17% and 79% of women of high school or college age will report binge-eating, with a clustering of prevalence rates between 45% and 60%.[64,69,88,152,153,158, 15,364,365,369,370, 371,373,398] The prevalence for men is similar, with a range of 38% to 62%.[152,364,365,369,371,373] Therefore, what is perceived as binge-eating by young men and women in the population at large is quite common, although this behavior probably is quite different from the behavior of most bulimic individuals.

How common is binge-eating in bulimia nervosa? Since binge-eating is required for the diagnosis, most reported series indicate that 100% of the patients have problems with binge-eating. Although the prevalence of self-reported binge-eating appears to be quite high in both patient and non-patient samples, the self-reported frequencies of the behavior are generally quite different. For example in the study by Pyle and colleagues of 1355 college freshman, only 2.4% reported daily binge-eating,[373] and the daily rate in a survey by Johnson and colleagues was 4%.[215] Therefore although perceived binge-eating is prevalent, it is infrequent in nonclinical populations compared to the frequency of this behavior in patients with bulimia nervosa, most of whom report daily binge-eating.

What actually constitutes binge-eating? The research group with which I work previously reported data on self-monitored binge-eating behavior in a series of outpatients who kept records of their eating prior to treatment.[312] The mean duration of binge-eating episodes in this group was 1.18 hours (range 15 minutes to 8 hours), with a mean number of binge-eating episodes a week of 11.7 and a mean amount of time spent binge-eating each week of 13.7 hours. The self-reported range of kilocalories ingested per eating binge ranged from 1200 to 11,500, with a mean of 3,415. Johnson and associates reported similar figures with an average estimated binge ingestion of 4,800 kilocalories.[212] Rosen and associates reported a mean intake during binge-eating episodes of 1,459 ± 1,172 in a series of 20 normal-weight female bulimics who kept eating records.[387] Also, our research group reported monitored binge-eating and vomiting behavior in a series of six bulimic women hospitalized on a research ward.[387] In this group of patients, the mean kilocalories ingested per binge-eating episode were 4,394 (range 1,436 to 8,585). Taken together, these studies, which have employed self-report or direct monitoring, suggest that there is considerable variability as to what constitutes an eating binge, but for the most part bulimic individuals consume a large amount of food, usually far in excess of the amount most people would consider simply overeating.

Rosen and associates reported that, while binge-eating, patients consume foods that are considered primarily snack or dessert foods.[387] In our outpatient survey, the most commonly ingested foods were ice cream, bread/toast, candy, doughnuts, and soft drinks.[312] Several authors also have recently looked at the macronutrient content of foods eaten during eating binges, and their results have been fairly consistent in indicating that bulimic individuals usually consume foods similar to those ingested by nonbulimic women in the same age group, with the caveat that binge foods are on average slightly higher in fat and slightly lower in protein compared to the typical diet of young women.[246,305] Although clinical lore suggests that binge-eating is typified by high carbohydrate intake, the monitored eating studies have not found this to be true overall, although it is clearly true for some patients.

Self-Induced Vomiting

Several studies that have examined the prevalence of bulimia and bulimia nervosa have included detailed questions about self-induced vomiting. Some have surveyed high school women and others college women.

In our survey of 1,355 freshman college students, 7.3% admitted to having self-induced vomiting, but only 0.9% of the sample did so on a daily basis.[373] In the 1981 Johnson and associates survey, 10.3% admitted to self-inducing vomiting, 1.6% on a daily basis. The results of these studies suggests that, relative to binge-eating, self-reported, self-induced vomiting is rare among women in this age group.[215] However, the prevalence of self-induced vomiting in women with bulimia nervosa ranges from 53.1% to 94.1% across the various reported studies, and in most of these studies the majority of bulimic patients also report a high frequency of self-induced vomiting, a finding seen very infrequently in surveys of young women in the general population.[99,102,135,216, 300,371,372] An example would be our survey of 275 outpatient bulimic women, 64% of whom reported a frequency of vomiting of several times a day, with an additional 8.1% reporting a frequency of once a day.[300] This suggests that self-induced vomiting is both quite prevalent and quite frequent among bulimic women, and that the presence of frequent self-induced vomiting should strongly suggest a diagnosis of an eating disorder.

For most patients with bulimia nervosa, self-induced vomiting either begins at about the same time as binge-eating, or follows the development of binge-eating by weeks, months, or years.[61] Only in a very small number does the vomiting develop first.[303] Early in the course of the illness, most bulimic individuals self-induce vomiting by stimulating their gag reflex mechanically, using a toothbrush, an eating utensil, or their hand;

however, many eventually learn to vomit reflexly without mechanical stimulation, and there is some indication that the gag reflex may decrease in intensity during chronic bulimia nervosa.[380] Some will ingest a large amount of fluid toward the end of the binge-eating episode to facilitate vomiting. Since there are medical conditions, such as Zenker's diverticulum, that can cause vomiting,[75] it is important to find out whether the patient self-induces the vomiting.

Laxative Abuse

The prevalence of laxative misuse has also been studied among young women in general and among patients with bulimia nervosa in particular. Although several prevalence studies have included questions concerning laxative use, in most it is difficult to know whether laxatives were actually abused or simply used for constipation in a responsible manner. In our survey of 1,355 college freshman, 10.4% reported laxative usage and 0.5% reported using laxatives on a daily basis,[373] while Johnson and associates found that 7.3% of high school girls reported laxative usage, 1% on a daily basis.[215]

However, laxative abuse is quite common among patients with bulimia nervosa. In our original report we noted that 53% of 34 patients reported having misused laxatives for weight control.[371] Subsequent reports by our group and others have indicated that between 18.8% and 75% of patients with bulimia nervosa report laxative misuse, and, as with vomiting, the frequency of usage is also quite high in most reports.[102,216,300,371,372] In our series of 275 patients, 19.7% admitted to using laxatives at least once a day for weight control, and 10% admitted using laxatives several times a day.[300]

It is often difficult to pinpoint the precipitating event for laxative abuse, but the general pattern is that patients with bulimia nervosa ingest these substances after a binge-eating episode to lose weight, feel thinner, and "get rid" of the food they have eaten.[254,255,294,295] Although all classes of laxatives can be misused, the class most often implicated is the class of stimulant laxatives, particularly those containing phenolpthalein, examples being Ex-Lax® and Correctol®, or those containing anthraquinones, an example being Senokot®. If adequate amounts of these laxatives are ingested, several hours later the individual will experience an abrupt, watery diarrhea. The fluid loss from the diarrhea engenders a sense of weight loss, causing the user to believe that she is really thinner, or at least has rid herself of the excess calories she ingested during the eating binge. However, the available literature suggests that any caloric absorption prevented by laxative misuse is minimal;[30] it is the fluid loss that accounts for the weight loss. Lacey and Gibson demonstrated the ineffectiveness of laxative abuse by showing that patients who self-induced vomiting ate significantly more during eating binges yet weighed less than those who used laxatives.[254,255] Despite their ineffectiveness, the use of laxatives tend to lead to further usage, since the individual develops reflex fluid retention in response to the laxative-induced dehydration. Therefore, a day or so after ingesting the laxatives the individual gains weight and may feel edematous. This may lead to repeat laxative usage. Over time, tolerance to the laxatives develops, and the dosage has to be increased. It is not uncommon to find individuals with bulimia nervosa who are taking 20, 40, 60, or more laxatives a day. Although many of these individuals believe that they are thus losing weight, what they are actually doing is gaining and losing fluid, and the use of the laxatives actually preordains the fluid retention.

Diuretic Abuse

Analogous to the situation with laxatives, we know little about the prevalence of diuretic misuse in the general population. The picture is also complicated by the fact that both prescription and over-the-counter diuretics are available. Our survey found that 6.2% of female college students admitted to using diuretics and 2.1% admitted to doing so on a daily basis,[373] while Johnson and associates found that 4.1% of high school students admitted to using diuretics, 1.2% on a daily basis.[215] How much of this use actually constituted abuse is unclear. There is also some evidence that patients seen in other contexts, such as those who consult physicians for fluid retention, may be misusing diuretics and may actually have an eating disorder.[309] This may be particularly true of individuals with "idiopathic edema" who seek diuretic prescriptions.[310]

The percentage of bulimic patients who use diuretics ranges from 33.9% to 40.6% in various studies.[102,216,300] In our data, 10.2% had used diuretics on at least a daily basis for weight control, again suggesting an association between diuretic use and bulimia nervosa.

Diuretics are available in a wide variety of over-the-counter and prescription formulations.[58,112,172,400] The relative prevalence of abuse of over-the-counter versus prescription diuretics is unclear. Most of the cases of diuretic abuse that have appeared in the literature involve the more potent prescription diuretics.[80] This is not meant to imply that abuse of over-the-counter prescriptions is not as much of a problem since these individuals are much less likely to come to medical attention, such abuse may only be a less visible problem.

Some patients with bulimia nervosa ingest diuretics after binge-eating in an attempt to lose weight. As with laxitive use, they may develop a sense of having lost weight, owing to the resultant dehydration; but what they have actually lost is fluid. The effect is temporary, and the individual may then get into the cycle of using the diuretic to ameliorate the reflex fluid retention that it induces.

Diet Pills

Most of the diet pill usage in patients with bulimia nervosa appears to involve over-the-counter diet pills, which usually contain phenylpropanolamine.[309] Of the surveys we have mentioned, only Johnson and associates reported data on diet pill usage.[215] In their sample of female high school students, 13% had used diet pills, 3.2% on a daily basis. Recently, Killen and colleagues reported that 8.3% of female 10th grade students reported using diet pills.[241,242] How much of this usage occurred in individuals with eating disorders is unclear. However, the prevalence of diet pill usage reported in patients with bulimia nervosa is variable but often quite high, ranging from 4.6% to 50.2% in various samples.[102,216,300] For example, in our series 25.2% of patients reported having used diet pills at least once a day for a period of time during the course of their illness.[300]

We recently solicited information about diet pill usage from a series of 100 women who were evaluated for bulimia nervosa in our clinic (unpublished data). Twenty-six reported having used diet pills during the month prior to evaluation: 8 several times a day, 10 several times a week, and 8 at a lower frequency. The most commonly used agents were Dexatrim® (92.3%), Dietac®(11.5%), and Accutrim® (7.7%). The particular drugs available will depend on the country or region.

The logistics of diet pill usage has not been adequately investigated. Patients may take one or more than one of the pills daily as a way of suppressing their appetite. However, only rarely do patients with eating disorders ingest large amounts of diet pills, or use "street" amphetamines.

Other Reported Behaviors

Rumination

Rumination—the regurgitation, chewing and reswallowing of food—has been described as a feeding problem among infants and children. However, recently there have been reports of this behavior occurring in adults as well. Although one report suggested that this behavior is probably benign,[273] other work suggests that the presence of rumination is highly suggestive of an underlying diagnosis of bulimia nervosa.[259] Fairburn and Cooper reported that 7 of 35 patients with bulimia nervosa reported habitual rumination, with 4 ruminating each day.[103]

Chewing and Spitting out Food

Fairburn and Cooper reported that 13 out of the 35 patients in one series indicated that they chewed and spit out food as part of their disorder, and 7 reported doing so on a regular basis.[103] In our series of 275 patients, 64.5% reported this behavior, although we did not collect frequency data.[300] Most recently we compared a series of 20 patients who chewed and spit out food on a regular basis at a frequency of at least several times a week with a control group of bulimic women who did not report this behavior.[315] The two groups were quite similar in terms of other associated problems. The significance of chewing and spitting out food as a symptom of bulimia nervosa is unclear.

Fasting

Many patients with bulimia nervosa eventually experience crowding out of normal eating behavior as the illness progresses, and many eat little, if at all, when not binge-eating. However, 24-hour fasting is relatively rare.[300]

Exercise

As with anorexia nervosa, excessive exercise can be a part of the syndrome, and this possibility should be addressed in each patient's history.[451] However, to my knowledge, the prevalence of excessive exercise and the patterns of exercise in this population have not been adequately studied. Developing a regular pattern of healthy exercise is important to the process of recovery, as will be discussed in the section on treatment.

Enemas

A small subgroup of these patients abuse enemas in an attempt to get rid of food and lose weight.[74,300]

3

Associated Problems

Bulimia nervosa is frequently accompanied by other forms of psychopathology and other associated difficulties. We turn now to a discussion of these areas.

Depression

There is much evidence to suggest a strong link between these disorders.[171,432, 458] Much of this work has been published by Pope, Hudson, and their colleagues at Maclean Hospital, who have been particularly interested in this association. The relationship with depression is important to our understanding of bulimia nervosa and quite controversial,[72, 189,265,303,447,462,474] (as is the relationship between anorexia nervosa and depression)[50,89] and we will discuss it in some depth.

First, there is an apparently high rate of depression among patients with bulimia nervosa. Rarely this depression reaches psychotic proportions.[186] Several of the studies which have employed structural assessment techniques to establish the prevalence of depression among bulimic patients are summarized in table 7. As can be seen, the rates are surprisingly high, given our knowledge of the base prevalence of affective disorders. However, one must also note that not all patients with bulimia nervosa are significantly depressed. In addition, Cooper and Fairburn have demonstrated that the depressive symptoms of depressed patients with and without bulimia nervosa often differ, which suggests divergent mechanisms.[70]

The obvious question is, what is causing what? Does bulimia nervosa engender the development of depression, or should depression be regard-

Table 7. Affective Disorders Diagnoses in Patients with Bulimia Nervosa Using Structured Interviews

Authors/Year	Instrument	N	Prevalence of Depression
Herzog et al./1984	RDC	55	24% current major depressive disorder
Walsh et al./1985	RDC		73% lifetime major depressive disorder
			29% current major depressive disorder
Hudson et al./1987			
Outpatients BN	DIS	50	59% lifetime major depressive disorder
Remitted BN	DIS	21	47% lifetime major depressive disorder
Controls	DIS	28	29% lifetime major depressive disorder

ed as a primary causal factor for the development of bulimia nervosa? A third hypothesis is that a common factor, perhaps some biological diathesis, preordains a risk for the development of both types of problems. How can we sort out the relative merit of these hypotheses, all of which are plausible? One approach is to examine the temporal association between the development of depression and bulimia nervosa. Put simply, what comes first? Here, again, the data are unclear.[101,192,257] Our group has published a paper showing that late onset bulimia nervosa appears to correlate with previous problems of depression, whereas early onset bulimia nervosa patients are less likely to have significant problems of depression.[302] Regardless of the causal direction, the comorbidity problem is significant.

Second, there also appears to be a familial relationship between these two conditions. Various research groups have published family history studies of bulimia nervosa, and the majority of these studies suggests a familial relationship between that condition and affective disorder, demonstrating that an individual with bulimia nervosa is more likely to have relatives with affective disorder than someone who does not have bulimia nervosa.[29,183,184, 187,188,192,420,452] This suggests some common diathesis for both conditions. However, one study has found that most of the relatives with depression cluster in the families of those bulimic individuals who are depressed themselves, suggesting that it is the depression and not the bulimia nervosa that accounts for the family loading.[424]

A third way to examine the relationship between depression and bulimia nervosa is to look at biological parameters. As reviewed by Hudson, Pope, and their colleagues,[183,184] there are certain common physiological changes in patients with bulimia nervosa that resemble those seen in depressed patients, including lack of suppression on the dexamethasone-suppression test. However, recent research suggests that the pathophysiology of the lack of suppression is different in these two conditions. Lack of suppression on the DST is probably attributable to poor absorption of dexamethasone in patients with bulimia nervosa, while disinhibition of the hypothalmic-pituitary-adrenal axis appears to be involved in the lack of suppression depression.[457] This is reviewed in the chapter on psychobiology.

Another observation that suggests a commonality between bulimia nervosa and affective disorders is the fact that patients with both conditions often respond favorably to antidepressant medication. There is now a large published literature on this, and the data from the studies are summarized in the chapter on psychopharmacology. However, response to antidepressants must be viewed as nonspecific, in that antidepressants are used for conditions that are not necessarily related to depression, such as blocking panic attacks in patients who are not depressed but who have anxiety disorders, and in the control of pain.

In summary, we cannot state with any assurance why there is such a high rate of comorbidity between these two types of disorders. However, clinically the comorbidity is quite important, and it does offer some very interesting leads for research.

Personality Disorders

The relationship between certain personality disorders or traits, including the personality disorder system described in DSM-III-R, and bulimia nervosa, is at this point controversial.[25,349] Two primary approaches have been taken to examine these relationships. First, some research has attempted to examine the personality styles or traits of patients with bulimia nervosa.[71] Second, other studies have used questionnaires or interviews designed to assess DSM-III or DSM-III-R Axis II disorders in patients with bulimia nervosa. The results of these studies have yielded widely disparate findings, as is summarized in table 8.[145,214,271,358]

As can be seen, different authors have found markedly different rates for Axis II pathology. For example, the work of Johnson and colleagues suggests a very high prevalence for borderline personality disorder in individuals with bulimia nervosa, while the work of Hudson and colleagues suggests the opposite. How do we resolve these discrepancies? One possi-

Table 8. Bulimia Nervosa and Borderline Personality Disorder

Year	Authors	N	Instrument	Percentage Positive
1983	Gwirtsman	18	Clinical	44%
1987	Levine and Hyler	24	PDQ, clinical	25%
1987	Hudson et al.	52	Diagnostic interview for borderline	2%
1988	Johnson et al.	95	Borderline syndrome index	45%

ble explanation is the nature and limitations of the instruments involved. Although the instruments that have come to the fore in assessing Axis II pathology have shed some light on the rather difficult area of personality assessment, it remains debatable whether or not they actually identify personality constructs that are stable over time. The results may reflect more the effects of the stress induced by the psychiatric and medical aspects of the disorder rather than stable personality configurations. It has been my experience, and others have noted this as well, that many patients with bulimia nervosa at initial assessment look as though they may have a significant personality disorder, appearing very dysfunctional in their relationships and to be using fairly primitive, immature defense mechanisms.[104,343] Later, after their eating behavior is brought under control, they look considerably healthier as to their overall adjustment and level of maturity. Therefore, pending the development of more precise measurements and more of an understanding as to what actually constitutes personality pathology, I think we must keep an open mind about the relationship between eating disorders and personality disorders.

Alcohol/Drug Abuse

Russell, in his original description of bulimia nervosa in 1979, noted that many patients with bulimia nervosa also have problems with drugs.[390] Subsequent research has documented this association.[16,38,44,223] In 1986 our group reported that of 275 women evaluated for bulimia in an outpatient clinic, 30.4% gave a history of having had problems with alcohol or other drugs, 23% had a history of alcohol or drug abuse, and 17.7% had previously been in alcohol/drug abuse treatment. These are very high rates, given that the mean age of this group of patients was 24, and most had not lived through the age of risk for developing alcohol and drug problems.[300] Other research has substantiated this problem. For example, Bulik[46] recently reported that the rate of alcohol and drug abuse problems was significantly higher among 35 women presenting for treatment with bulimia nervosa compared to age- and sex-matched controls. Also, Jonas and colleagues reported a very high rate of eating disorders among female callers to the National Cocaine Hotline.[222]

Similar research has shown the same comorbidity problem for women who present with alcohol and drug abuse problems.[193,256] Our group found that the rate of self-reported pathological eating behavior, such as daily binge-eating and daily self-induced vomiting, was significantly higher among women with alcohol and drug abuse problems than among controls, and women with alcohol and drug abuse problems are more than twice as likely to satisfy operationalized DSM-III criteria for bulimia nervosa as well.

Several papers[49,154,155] have summarized some of the behavioral similarities between alcohol/drug abuse and eating disorders. These include the observation that both types of problems involve the misuse of a substance, craving the substance, and using the substance for mood-altering effects and as a means of coping and avoiding unpleasant situations. Both also involve repeated attempts at control of usage, and resulting financial, physical, and psychological problems. Also, patients with the dual diagnosis of bulimia nervosa and alcohol/drug abuse problems are at higher risk for other problems, including abuse of diuretics and more serious social impairment than women who only have bulimia nervosa. They are also more likely to report a history of suicidal and/or stealing behavior, and to have been hospitalized for psychiatric problems.[157]

As with depression, there is clearly a problem of comorbidity. However, the exact reason for this comorbidity remains unclear. Some have suggested that bulimia nervosa and alcohol/drug abuse problems should be classified as related addictions.[38] However, not all patients with bulimia nervosa develop alcohol/drug abuse problems despite the increased prevalence, and there are some significant differences between the two conditions. Those differences have serious implications for treatment, most importantly, is that individuals with bulimia nervosa need to eat. They cannot simply avoid the substance of abuse (food) as patients with alcohol and drug abuse problems can.

Some, but not all, studies have also suggested a familial relationship between alcohol/drug abuse problems and bulimia nervosa.[188,420,452] Most recently, Hudson and his colleagues[187] demonstrated that the rate of alcohol and drug abuse problems was significantly higher among the first-degree relatives of individuals with bulimia nervosa than among those of age-matched controls.

Body Image Disturbance

The DSM-III-R criteria require preoccupation with issues of shape and weight. It is clear that many women with bulimia nervosa are obsessed with these issues, and many have a disturbed body image.[27,65,199,338,366,442] However, it is less clear whether patients with bulimia nervosa have more of a problem with distorted body image than other young women. This topic has recently been reviewed by Meerman and Vandereycken,[289] including the size estimation and distortion image techniques that have been used. Taken together, this literature remains controversial.

Social Impairment and Low Self-Esteem

Generally the course of bulimia nervosa is complicated by an increasing degree of social impairment.[92,164,167,169,209,231,336,343] This is particularly true of those patients with a concomitant affective disorder or substance-use disorder.[157] This impairment can manifest itself in several ways. Many times patients experience considerable social isolation. They must isolate themselves to binge-eat; however, many of them develop social isolation secondarily for other reasons. The untruthfulness that characterizes this disorder can affect relationships adversely. Bulimic individuals frequently have to cancel appointments or dates they have made because of the decision to binge-eat and vomit. Perhaps owing to the depression and the nutritional disturbances, many find that they do not perform well in school or on the job. In one study, bulimic women demonstrated about the same degree of social impairment as a matched group of women with alcoholism.[209] In 1986, Lacey and colleagues reported data on adjustment in 50 female bulimia nervosa subjects.[253] The women reported marked doubts about their own femininity, poor relationships and much conflict with their parents, and poor peer relationships. Butterfield and Laclair reported that patients with bulimia nervosa tend to denigrate themselves.[49] Social impairment, low self-esteem, negativity, and the sense of personal ineffectiveness that characterize this disorder[397,454,465] have obvious ramifications for treatment. A recent report by Fairburn and colleagues indicates that self-esteem is an important predictor of success in treatment.[107]

Family Problems

Clinical observations suggest that there are significant problems in many of the families of bulimic patients, and family therapy is probably the treatment of choice for some patients, particularly younger adolescents.[248,249,343,449] What is less clear is whether these problems predispose to, or are caused by, the illness. Johnson and Flach in 1985 compared family data from 105 patients diagnosed as having DSM-III bulimia with data on 86 control families.[211] The bulimic families scored lower on cohesiveness, demonstrated a higher level of conflict, and in general evidenced lack of emphasis on independence and assertiveness in the children. Sights and Richards[408] found, in studying families of bulimic patients, that the mothers tended to be more controlling than the mothers in control families. Garner and colleagues compared the families of normal-weight bulimic patients to those with both restricting and bulimic anorexia nervosa families.[125] They found more familial pathology in both the normal-weight and anorectic bulimic groups. However, it is less clear if there is a specific type of family system that seems to engender, or perhaps results from, having a bulimic child. The possibility of a genetic diathesis for bulimia nervosa has not been adequately investigated; however, concordance for this disorder has been reported in a pair of monozygotic twins.[226]

Other Problems

Several other problem behaviors have been linked either anecdotally or experimentally with bulimia nervosa, including self-injurious behavior such as self-cutting,[21,415,437] suicidal behavior, stealing,[129,130] and general problems with impulsivity.[399,441,466,472] How closely these problems correlate with the diagnosis of bulimia nervosa is unclear, but some have speculated that a significant subgroup of individuals with bulimia nervosa have a more global "loss-of-control" problem, which manifests itself not just in eating behavior, but in other areas of functioning as well. Clearly though, these other problems do not characterize all patients with bulimia nervosa. Research also suggests an association between eating disorders and a past history of sexual abuse, a finding with important therapy implications.[342]

4

Assessing Patients with Bulimia Nervosa

This chapter is devoted to a discussion of diagnostic interview techniques that can be used to identify individuals with bulimia nervosa. Some of this material has been included, in a different form, in a published patient self-report database, the Eating Disorders Questionnaire, developed at the University of Minnesota.[301]

The information presented here should be included in a thorough evaluation history of an individual with an eating disorder. Although the suggested interview format is suitable for patients with other eating problems, it is designed specifically for bulimic individuals.

Before turning to the specifics of the interview, I will make some general comments. Some individuals who present for evaluation for eating disorders have never discussed their eating problems with anyone before, and it may be difficult for them to talk freely about many of their behaviors. Therefore, although it is certainly useful to encourage patients to present as much material as possible spontaneously using an open-ended approach, at some point the interviewer should shift to direct questioning and, in a supportive nonjudgmental way, ask about all the potential associated problems. Not to do so may spare the patient some initial embarrassment, but will permit her to continue to have "secrets," about which she will probably feel guilty, and also will prevent the development of a complete, realistic treatment plan. For example, if the patient is using laxatives or ipecac, behavior the interviewer needs to know about, she may not volunteer this information except on careful questioning.

A direct, forthright approach is best because it communicates to the patient that the interviewer is familiar with such problems, has encountered them before, is not going to be surprised or offended, and is open to discuss such issues.

Since patients with bulimia nervosa are at times dishonest about what they have been doing (although many have decided to be honest about their behavior when they come for treatment), the interviewer must always suspect that associated problems may be present.

The form in which questions are asked is important. A question such as "You don't use laxatives, do you?" is much less likely to illicit useful information than the query "Do you now or have you ever used laxatives for weight control?"

What follows is an outline of the information that should be included in a complete history. The sequence is unimportant. Patients rarely present information in a logical sequence, but all of these areas need to be covered if the interviewer wants a clear picture of the patient's problems.

  I. Demographic Information
    A. Sex
    B. Age
    C. Race
    D. Religious affiliation
    E. Marital status
    F. Present primary role (wage-earner? student?)
    G. Educational background
    H. Current occupation

 II. Weight History
    A. Current weight and height?
    B. Desired ("ideal") weight?
    C. What does the patient think would be a "healthy" weight for her?
    D. Highest adult weight? At what age?
    E. Lowest adult weight? At what age?
    F. Does the patient have frequent weight fluctuations? If so, how large?
    G. Highest weight between ages 12 and 18? At what age?
    H. Lowest weight between ages 12–18? At what age?
    I. Is the individual involved in an occupation or participating in a sport which requires a certain weight? (e.g. ballet, wrestling, cheerleading, dance line)?

J. How would a two-pound weight gain affect the patient's feeling about herself?

K. How would a two-pound weight loss affect the patient's feeling about herself?

L. Does the individual fear becoming fat, and if so, how strong is this fear?

M. Is this patient dissatisfied with the way her body is proportioned?

N. Which body parts are perceived in a positive way and which in a negative way?

O. How often does this patient weigh herself?

III. Dieting Behavior

A. How many meals does the patient eat each day (not including binge-eating, snacking, or meals followed by vomiting)?

B. How many snacks does she eat each day?

C. What are the meals and snacks like? (It is useful to have patients go through and describe a typical 24-hour food intake pattern.)

D. Does this patient attempt to avoid certain foods? Which ones?

E. Has this individual ever been on a diet?

F. At what age did the patient first begin to restrict her food intake?

G. Has the patient been dieting recently?

H. What types of diets has this individual tried? (Some examples follow.)

  1. Weight Watchers®
  2. Supervised dieting
  3. Unsupervised dieting
  4. Very low-calorie diets
  5. Protein-sparing fasts
  6. TOPS®
  7. Liquid protein diet
  8. HCG shots
  9. Behavior modification
  10. Psychotherapy
  11. Hypnosis
  12. Overeaters Anonymous

IV. Binge-Eating Behavior

    A. Has the patient had periods of time when she would eat a large amount of food in a short period of time (binge-eating)?

    B. What are the characteristics of the patient's binge-eating behavior?

        1. Does she consume a large amount of food?

        2. Does she eat rapidly?

        3. Does she feel out of control when binge-eating?

        4. Does she feel miserable, annoyed, or depressed after an eating binge?

        5. Does she feel that she has uncontrollable urges to eat?

        6. Does she isolate herself while binge-eating?

        7. How long do the binge-eating episodes last?

    C. When is the patient most likely to binge-eat?

        1. In the evening (most common pattern)?

        2. Anytime?

    D. Where is the patient most likely to binge-eat?

        1. At home (most common place)?

        2. In her car (not an uncommon second choice)?

    E. How old was the patient when she first started binge-eating?

    F. What is the longest period of time she has been able to control her binge-eating?

    G. What foods does this patient eat while binge-eating? Does she eat these foods when not binge-eating?

    H. Has she noticed a relationship between binge-eating and her menstrual cycle?

    I. How uncomfortable is the patient with her binge-eating behavior? Is she motivated to change it?

    J. How often has she been binge-eating recently?

V. Purging Behavior

    A. Has the patient engaged in self-induced vomiting to rid herself of food or to lose weight?

    B. How old was she when she first engaged in this behavior?

    C. Has she ever been able to control the behavior for a period of time?

    D. How frequently has she been self-inducing vomiting lately?

E. Which of the behaviors came first — binge-eating or vomiting — or did they start at about the same time?

F. Has the patient ever used laxatives to control weight or "get rid" of food?

   1. How old was she when she first began using laxatives?

   2. How long has she used laxatives for weight control?

   3. What laxatives does she use?

   4. How many laxatives does she take when she uses them?

VI. Other Weight-Control Measures

A. Does this patient use diet pills in an attempt to control her weight?

   1. Which ones?

   2. How many a day?

   3. For how long?

   4. Prescription or over-the-counter?

B. Has this patient ever chewed and spit out food without swallowing to avoid food intake or to lose weight? For how long?

C. Has this individual ever ruminated food? How often?

D. Does this patient ever use water pills or diuretics to lose weight?

   1. Which ones?

   2. For how long?

   3. At what dosage?

   4. Prescription or over-the-counter?

(In general, it is good to have both durations and frequencies for all the various behaviors we have mentioned, including binge-eating, vomiting, and use of laxatives, diet pills, and diuretics.)

E. Has this patient ever used the drug ipecac to stimulate vomiting?

   1. How many times?

   2. At what dosage?

VII. Exercise

A. How frequently does she exercise?

B. How long are exercise sessions?

C. Why is she exercising?

      1. Fitness?

      2. To lose weight?

      3. Other (stipulate)?

VIII. Other Behaviors

    A. Has this individual ever had a problem with alcohol or drug abuse?

      1. Which substances?

      2. For how long?

      3. What is the current usage pattern?

    B. Does this person have a history of suicide attempts? Self-injurious behavior (cutting herself, hitting, or burning herself)?

    C. Has this person been involved in stealing?

      1. What sorts of items?

      2. Beginning at what age?

      3. Ever arrested?

      4. What are the reasons she steals?

IX. Affective Symptoms

    A. It is best to go through a complete list of possible depressive symptoms, including the following:

      1. Has the individual had sadness or depressed moods?

      2. Sleep disturbance?

      3. Problems with concentration?

      4. Problems with memory?

      5. Decreased energy, fatigue?

      6. Suicidal ideas?

    B. Has the person been treated previously for depression?

    C. What does the pattern of depression suggest?

      1. Dysthymia?

      2. Recurrent major depressive disorder? Single episode?

      3. Active or in remission?

      4. Secondary problem to the bulimia nervosa?

X. Menstrual History

    A. Age of onset of menstruation?

    B. Any periods of amenorrhea or oligomenorrhea?

    C. Regularity of menses since the onset of bulimia nervosa?

    D. Has the patient menstruated in the last three months?

XI. Past Psychiatric History

    A. It is important to ask questions concerning all the major diagnostic groupings. For example:

        1. Does the patient meet criteria for obsessive-compulsive disorder or other anxiety disorders?

        2. Is there evidence of an Axis II problem?

(The usual psychiatric interview can be used to examine for other types of psychopathology. It is useful to specifically examine what types of treatments the patient has had before and what her responses were, particularly to antidepressants or psychotherapy.)

    B. Has the patient ever been hospitalized before?

        1. For what reason?

        2. For how long?

    C. Medical History

    The history should also include other elements of the standard medical history, including a thorough past medical history, and history of allergic problems (drug or otherwise) and previous medications, with particular attention to over-the-counter drugs that can be abused by patients with bulimia nervosa.

    D. Family History

    A careful family history should be obtained concerning other forms of psychopathology, obesity, and physical problems.

XII. Review of Systems

A review of systems should be pursued, including special attention to problems commonly encountered in patients with bulimia nervosa, such as weakness, low energy, dental problems, sali-' vary gland swelling, constipation, diarrhea, hematemesis, black tarry stools, fainting, sore throat, abdominal pain, edema.

XIII. Mental Status Examination

    A. A thorough mental status examination should also be included.

5

Medical Complications/
Medical Management

Bulimia nervosa is a more medically benign condition than anorexia nervosa, wherein most of the medical complications are attributed to starvation.[239] However, some physicians and therapists who work with eating disorders patients assume that this condition is not physically hazardous, underestimating the potential for complications. In this chapter, we will review the major medical complications of this disorder and offer guidelines for their assessment and management. For those interested, there are several additonal books and papers that offer much useful summary information on these complications.[39,82,59,134,292,318,431,477] The most important point of the chapter is that all patients with bulimia nervosa should be carefully assessed medically.

When thinking about the medical complications of bulimia nervosa, it is useful to remember that the complications result from the specific behaviors involved in the syndrome. For example, dental enamel erosion,[413] a common complication of this disorder, is directly attributable to vomiting, which exposes the surface of the teeth to the highly acidic gastric acid. Another example would be the electrolyte abnormalities that occur commonly in individuals with bulimia nervosa, which result from the vomiting and/or laxative abuse, and the attendant fluid depletion, as well as inadequate fluid intake.[313] Therefore, specific behaviors can result in specific complications that are, for the most part, readily reversible when the behaviors are interrupted.

Before turning to the signs and symptoms of this disorder, I have compiled a list of both the most common and most serious medical problems that can arise, and discussed their signs, symptoms, the associated X-ray

Table 9. An Overview of Medical Complications of Bulimia Nervosa.

Problem	Reason	Symptoms	Signs	X-ray/Laboratory	Management
Dehydration	Vomiting Laxatives Diuretics Fluid restriction	Dizziness Lightheadedness Weakness	Hypotension Tachycardia	Hemoconcentration (Serum osmo., hct.)	Encourage fluid intake Encourage ↓ vomiting laxatives diuretics
Salivary gland hypertrophy	Unclear	"Puffy cheeks" "Fat face"	Salivary gland swelling	Serius amylase	Rx Primary disorder
Dental enamel erosion	Vomiting	Tooth sensitivity Tooth erosion	Enamel erosion		Rx Vomiting Rinse, *not brush* after vomiting; Bicarbonate rinses
Metabolic alkalosis; Hypochloremia, Hypokalemia	Vomiting Laxatives Diuretics	Dizziness Weakness Muscle twitching Palpitations	Rare: arrythmias, clonus	Serum bicarb. Serum Cl,K EKG abnormalities	Encourage fluid intake Encourage ↓ vomiting laxatives diuretics
Metabolic acidosis	Laxatives			Serum bicarb.	Encourage ↓ laxatives
Gastric dilatation	Binge-eating	Severe abdominal pain; can't vomit	Distended abdomen	Enlarged gastric silouette	Attempt nasogastric decompression Surgery consult stat.
Gastric rupture	Binge-eating	Severe abdominal pain; guarding symptoms of shock	Rigid abdomen, shock	Free air under the diaphragm	Surgical emergency
Esophageal rupture	Vomiting	Chest, abdominal or back pain	Dissection of pain under the skin	Extravasation of contrast media on esophagram	Medical management vs surgical intervention

or laboratory findings, if any, and their management, in table 9. It may be useful to refer to this table as you read the chapter.

Patients with bulimia nervosa who are seen by physicians for physical problems or by therapists for other psychological symptoms may fail to report their eating problems. The single most important element in diagnosing bulimia nervosa is a high index of suspicion. Physicians and therapists who encounter patients in this age group should routinely consider this diagnosis and ask the appropriate questions, even if patients do not mention such problems spontaneously. There are also certain symptoms and signs that occur commonly among these patients that might suggest the diagnosis. We turn now to a discussion of these.

Physical Symptoms

Patients with bulimia nervosa frequently have physical complaints when they come for therapy. Two studies have systematically examined these complaints. Abraham and Beumont reported that the most common physical symptoms mentioned by a series of 32 bulimic patients were swelling of the hands and feet (69%), abdominal fullness (66%), fatigue (47%), headache (38%), and nausea (34%).[2] In a report of 275 women with bulimia, our group found the most commonly reported symptoms were weakness (84%); a "bloated" feeling (75%); "puffy cheeks," presumably secondary to salivary gland swelling, (50%); dental problems (37%); and finger callouses, presumably related to trauma to the dorsum of the hand caused by using the hand to mechanically stimulate the vomiting reflex. (27%).[300]

The results of these studies show that many women with bulimia will report physical complaints that are understandable given the involved behaviors.

Physical Signs

Unlike anorexia nervosa, where the emaciation of the patient usually alerts the clinician to the diagnosis, most patients with bulimia nervosa have few physical stigmata. However, there are certain signs, present on physical examination, that are of some utility.[142]

The most common sign is erosion of the dental enamel. This change was originally described in patients with anorexia nervosa,[200] but more recently has been found in bulimic patients who vomit.[62,178,218,413,479]

What is observed clinically is decalcification of the lingual, palatal, and posterior occlusal surfaces of the teeth. The erosion of the dental enamel is often particularly marked on the inside (toward the tongue) surface of the upper teeth.[413] The fillings or amalgams, which are relatively resistant to the gastric acid, eventually project above the surface of the enamel, which appears washed-out around them. In one recent study, the majority of bulimia patients who had been vomiting at least three times a week for four years showed evidence of this pattern on dental examination.[413] The changes are not hard to detect once the examiner knows what to look for and how to interpret the findings. A second clinical sign is hypertrophy of the salivary glands, particularly the parotid glands.[9,48,203,272,377,414,439] The swelling is usually bilateral and painless, but at times can be quite pronounced. The exact prevalence of this finding among bulimic women is unknown. it may be fairly common but, when only of modest proportions, difficult to recognize on physical examination. Clear clinical evidence on physical examination of salivary hypertrophy is present only in a minority of patients.

A third sign of diagnostic utility is scarring or callous formation on the back of the hand, caused by using the hand to self-induce vomiting. Originally described by Russell,[390] the lesions can vary from elongated superficial ulceration to hyperpigmented callouses or scarring.[224,401,483] To my knowledge researchers have not evaluated the prevalence of this sign or the course of this complication during the illness. However, it is my impression that these lesions are more common early in the course of the disorder, before patients have taught themselves to vomit reflexly. The dermatologic signs associated with eating disorders have recently been reviewed by Gupta and colleagues.[144]

Cardiovascular Complications

There are several possible cardiovascular complications of bulimia nervosa. The most common is dehydration, which develops secondary to vomiting or abusing laxatives or diuretics.[313] The associated intravascular fluid contraction can result in hypotension with lightheadedness, dizziness, or fainting. Also quite common, and again attributable to the associated behaviors, are electrolyte abnormalities, which secondarily can cause cardiovascular problems.[313] Electrolyte abnormalities will be reviewed in another section.

Another complicating behavior, which unfortunately may be a growing problem in this population of patients, is the misuse of ipecac as a way of stimulating vomiting. Ipecac is a drug that is available over-the-counter, and is marketed to induce emesis when individuals ingest dangerous substances.[5,114,319] The drug is a powerful emetic, and for this reason some individuals with eating disorders take the drug after eating as a way to induce vomiting and rid themselves of food. Although a causal relationship between the use of the drug and fatal cardiomyopathies has not been firmly established,[202] several case reports strongly suggest a link, and it is well documented that the drug can result in peripheral myopathies as well.[19,115,206,320] This will be discussed in more detail in a later section.

Recently, Johnson and associates reported increased rates of mitral valve prolapse in patients with bulimia nervosa compared to age-matched controls.[219] The significance of this finding is unclear.

Endocrine/Metabolism Complications

Several interesting endocrine and metabolic problems have been described in this population.[110,180,330] Most are discussed in the chapter on psychobiology. An apparent association between bulimia nervosa and diabetes mellitus has been reported.[170,181,194,389,435] Several cases of individuals with both diabetes mellitus and a concomitant eating disorder have appeared, and in several of these case reports it was well documented that the patient withheld insulin as a way of inducing glycosuria in order to rid herself of excess calories and promote weight loss. The exact prevalence of eating disorders among diabetic patients is unclear, but some preliminary work by Hudson and colleagues[195] suggests that this association is common. The authors systematically surveyed a series of diabetic patients. Although only 30% of those surveyed responded to the questionnaire, 35% of the responders met criteria for bulimia. It would appear that bulimia nervosa should be considered as a possibility in young diabetic women, particularly in those who pose difficult management problems.

Fluid and Electrolyte Abnormalities

Bulimia-associated behaviors, such as vomiting, laxative and diuretic abuse, and excessive exercise, can result in dehydration and volume contraction, as well as the loss of significant amounts of electrolytes such as sodium, potassium, and chloride.[309,313] The resultant electrolyte and acid/base disturbances are quite common. In a series of 168 patients seen in our clinic, 49% had at least a modest fluid or electrolyte abnormality, the most common being metabolic alkalosis suggested by an elevated serum bicarbonate (27%), hypochloremia (24%), hypokalemia (14%), and hyponatremia (5%).[313] It is important to emphasize the role of fluid loss in these abnormalities, since some clinicians assume such abnormalities result from the direct loss of electrolytes through vomiting. Volume depletion induced by vomiting and aggravated by fasting or diuretic or laxative abuse results in the generation of aldosterone, which promotes the loss of potassium through the kidneys. Because of the metabolic alkalosis, hydrogen ions shift into the extracellular fluid and, in exchange, potassium shifts into the cells. This sequence appears to account for the hypokalemia that is of such concern in many of these patients.

The picture is somewhat different in patients who have recently abused laxatives. Laxatives cause diarrhea, and diarrhea induces a loss of bicarbonate in the stool.[294, 295] Thus individuals who have recently abused laxatives may have a low serum bicarbonate, suggesting metabolic acidosis, an opposite picture to that described above. Therefore, alkalosis should suggest vomiting, laxative abuse, and volume depletion, while acidosis suggests recent misuse of laxatives.

Gastrointestinal

This area has recently been reviewed.[76] We have previously mentioned the problem of the salivary gland changes that are associated with bulimia nervosa. The mechanism of salivary gland hypertrophy is unclear, and various mechanisms have been implicated, including metabolic alkalosis, malnutrition, and high carbohydrate intake.[9,48,272,377,414,439] The results of the few reported biopsies indicate normal tissue or asymptomatic noninflammatory changes. Interestingly, this hypertrophy may persist for several months beyond normalization of eating behavior. Surgical treatment by superficial parotidectory has been reported;[24] however, the advisability of such a procedure in someone who is actively bulimic is clearly open to question.[377]

A laboratory finding that appears, at least in part, to be related to salivary gland hypertrophy is an elevation of serum amylase levels.[227] In a series from our clinic, 28% of patients had modest elevations of serum amlyase, although usually less than twice normal. Jacombs and Snyder reported that 15 of 24 patients in their series had elevated amylase levels.[203] These elevations were originally assumed to be salivary in origin, and Kaplan and associates documented that most bulimic patients with amylase elevations had isolated salivary isoamylase elevations.[227] However, Gwirtsman and associates found that both salivary and pancreatic isoenzymes contribute,[146] and Gavish and associates recently reported bulimia nervosa in association with relapsing hyperlipidemic pancreatitis,[127] suggesting the possibility of an associated problem with pancreatitis in a subgroup of these patients. Gilinsky and colleagues have also reported pancreatic abnormalities on CT scanning in patients with bulimia nervosa.[132] Therefore, the amylase elevation cannot be interpreted as always indicating salivary gland involvement, and a careful history is necessary to rule out pancreatitis involvement.

Esophageal or gastric perforation appears to be a rare but very serious complication of vomiting in bulimia nervosa.[204] It is impossible to know how many of the case reports of esophageal rupture reported in the literature involved bulimic individuals, since the diagnosis would not have been suspected until recently.[1,93,238,260,290,348,409] However, we have seen a case of esophageal rupture associated with vomiting and suspect that other cases unfortunately will be reported.

Another serious complication is gastric rupture. Saul and associates in 1981 reviewed the literature on this problem and noted that 11 of the cases in the literature had a diagnosis of anorexia nervosa.[395] In 10 additional cases there was a history of weight loss. These authors added the case of a 22-year-old woman who was well nourished but developed gastric infarction and perforation. Our research group also reported the case of a woman who developed gastric dilatation without rupture after binge-eating, and more recently other case reports have appeared.[1,35,93,292,317,348] The risk of gastric rupture is difficult to evaluate, but it appears to be a rare, albeit tragic complication of this disorder. The development of bulimia nervosa after gastric stapling for obesity also has been reported.[291]

Humphries and Shih reported that 60% of a series of 20 normal-weight bulimics had delayed gastric emptying—a finding that may help to explain the postprandial bloating that these women report.[198] However, Robinson and colleagues [382] found normal gastric emptying in 10 normal-weight bulimics.

Mediastinal Injuries

Several reports in the literature suggest a possible relationship between eating disorders and the development of pneumomediastinum.[7] Most of these reports have been of patients with anorexia nervosa; however, a recurrent theme in this literature is the possible role of vomiting in the development of this disorder, such as in the cases reported by Donley and Kemple,[85] Chatfield and colleagues,[57] and Bullimore and Cooke.[47] Fortunately this is a rare complication in these patients.

Neurological Complications

The nervous system has also been investigated in patients with bulimia nervosa for several reasons, including the fact that certain neural structures (particularly the hypothalamus) are involved in the control of eating behavior, and the knowledge that certain abnormalities of brain electrical activity can cause disordered eating.

Rau, Green, and their colleagues, in a series of papers, have examined the association between eating disorders, in particular the problem of compulsive eating, and electroencephalographic abnormalities. These authors have explored the central hypothesis that some neurophysiological abnormality might underlie certain types of eating problems.[137,374,376] A review by this group summarizing their results suggested that a majority of patients with compulsive eating disturbances had abnormal electroencephalograms. However, the abnormalities described are not accepted by all experts as indicative of significant pathology.[277,278,288,426,468] Our group reported a study of 25 patients who underwent sleep-deprived EEGs with NP leads.[304] All study tracings were read separately and blindly by two board-certified electroencephalographers, and 21 of the tracings were read as normal by both readers. We concluded that there did not appear to be a clear relationship between EEG abnormalities and bulimia nervosa, but that further work in this area appears to be indicated.

Although Lankenau and associates described no significant differences between the CT scanning results in the patients with bulimia nervosa compared to normal controls,[258] a recent larger study by Krieg and associates found evidence of atrophic changes on head CT in a subgroup of these patients.[251] The changes were less severe than those seen in anorexia nervosa, but significant compared to controls. The reversibility of this finding has yet to be studied. The significance of this finding, and its implications in terms of the cognitive functioning and nutritional status of patients with bulimia nervosa, remain to be explored.

It is important to remember that there are a number of potentially serious neurological problems that may present as disordered eating behavior and that must be considered in the differential diagnosis of bulimia nervosa. These include Huntington's chorea, binge-eating as a postictal phenomenon, and disordered eating as a result of space-occupying lesions such as tumors in the cerebral cortex or hypothalamus.[292,378]

Other Abnormalities

The case of a 28-year-old woman who presented with a bleeding diathesis and was found to have a vitamin-K-deficient coagulation factor deficiency has been reported.[331] As expected based on the other problems discussed, patients with bulimia nervosa can develop musculoskeletal problems (myopathies related to ipecac use or hypokalemia) or kidney problems (particularly hypokalemic nephropathy in those with chronic dehydration and chronic hypokalemia), but both of these complications are evidently rare. A case of "alcoholic hepatitis" in a nonalcoholic female with bulimia nervosa has been reported.[77]

Hunger and Taste

Hunger, satiety, and taste have also been studied in connection with bulimia nervosa. Jirik-Babb and Katz[208] have reported impaired taste perception in bulimia patients. The reason for this impairment is unclear, but may relate to the vomiting behavior. Drewnowski and colleagues have demonstrated that patients with bulimia nervosa tend to dislike high-fat foods and to prefer sweeter food stimuli compared to controls.[86,87] Also, bulimics report hunger sensations similar to normals, but have impaired satiety responses,[345] and after eating they tend to be irritable, tense, and depressed.[60]

Atypical Substances of Abuse

As discussed briefly in chapter 1 and in the discussion of medical complications, women with bulimia nervosa have a high risk of abusing several classes of compounds not usually considered drugs of abuse.[309] These include laxatives, diuretics, diet pills, and the over-the-counter emetic compound ipecac. In a previously reported survey of 275 bulimic women seen in our clinic,[300] 60.6% had used laxatives for weight control, 50.2% had used diet pills, and 33.9% had used diuretics during the course of their illness; this suggests that the misuse of these types of drugs is quite common in this population.

These drugs pose several risks. First, many of the patients who use them develop a strong psychological dependency on them and become convinced that they will gain weight if they discontinue their use. Second, the physical consequences of using these drugs can be quite damaging to several organ systems, and, in extreme cases, can be life endangering. Third, the use of these drugs often complicates treatment. It is particularly difficult to get outpatients to discontinue laxatives and diurectics because of the attendant fluid retention and weight gain. Therefore, it is important to examine each of these classes of drugs in some detail and discuss the management of patients who use them.

Laxatives

Commonly available laxatives are shown in table 10. Members of our group have previously reviewed some of the complications of laxative abuse,[294] which can be summarized as follows:

1. Constipation.[410] When patients have been chronically abusing these drugs, they commonly develop significant reflex hypofunctioning of the colon. This is particularly problematic when an attempt is made to discontinue the laxatives.
2. Cathartic colon.[243] Patients who have abused laxatives for long periods of time can develop permanent hypofunctioning of the colon.[379] In extreme cases, this has necessitated colostomy, although this appears to be very rare in younger bulimic patients.
3. Dehydration and electrolyte abnormalities.[78,261,292] Stimulant laxatives promote fluid loss through the intestine and volume contraction, leading to the development of secondary hyperaldosteronism and reflex peripheral edema, which is particularly problematic during laxative withdrawal. Laxative-induced diarrhea elevates the electrolyte content of the feces, resulting in hypochloremia and acidosis.
4. Other possible complications include GI bleeding,[467] weakness,[430] protein-losing gastroenteropathy,[410] pancreatic dysfunction,[270] and osteomalacia with pseudofractures.[116]

Table 10. Commonly Available Over-the-Counter Laxatives

Brand	Active Ingredient	Amount		Recommended* Dosage/Day
Correctol®	Tabs — yellow phenolpthalein	65	mg	1–2 tbsp
	docusate sodium	100	mg	
	Liquid — yellow phenolpthalein	65	mg	
Ex-Lax®	Yellow phenolpthalein	65	mg	1–2
Feen-a-Mint Gum®	Yellow phenolpthalein	79.2	mg	1–2
Feen-a-Mint Pills®	Yellow phenolpthalein	65	mg	1–2
	Docusate sodium	100	mg	
Nature's Remedy®	Cascara sagrada	150	mg	2
	Aloe	100	mg	

*Recommended package dosage.

Laxative withdrawal is difficult for most patients, many of whom experience significant fluid retention and constipation.[67,140] General guidelines to follow in withdrawing patients from stimulant laxatives include the following:

1. The laxative should be discontinued abruptly. There is no evidence that gradually tapering the drug will help the patient; if anything, this may prolong the agony and the problem with reflex constipation.
2. The patient needs to continue to maintain an adequate fluid intake to prevent further constipation. Many patients will restrict their fluid intake because of the edema. This is counter-therapeutic, in that it makes it less likely for them to have bowel movements. It is preferable to restrict sodium intake as a way of minimizing the amount of reflex edema.
3. It is important that patients be educated that they need to have regular bowel movements and that, if they do not have a bowel movement for three, four, or five days, they should contact the therapist. For those with protracted constipation, Metamucil® and/or lactulose seem to be useful short-term agents.
4. The addition of bran to the diet and/or the use of a high-fiber diet is recommended.
5. Regular physical exercise will help to regulate bowel functioning.

Diet Pills

These medications, summarized in table 11, have been a source of considerable debate in the medical community.[79,262,393] They do indeed induce weight loss on a short-term basis in individuals who are overweight,[8,139] but their safety and efficacy has not been evaluated in normal-weight individuals or with chronic usage. There are several anecdotal reports about side effects and toxicity that are of concern, including reports of elevated blood pressure, renal failure, seizures, and adverse neurological sequelae.[20,63,84,111,217,240,263,333,404] The management of diet pill usage is to get the patient to withdraw from the drug as quickly as possible.

Diuretics

There are several other medical related considerations to diuretic abuse. One is pseudo-Bartter's syndrome.[311,388,394,436] Bartter's syndrome is a renal disorder characterized by hypokalemia, alkalosis, elevated serum renin and aldosterone, normal blood pressure, and hyperplasia of the juxtaglomerular apparatus of the kidney.[15] The etiology is unknown, but appears to involve a problem with chloride reabsorption in the loop of Henle. All of the symptoms of Bartter's syndrome can be mimicked by diuretic abuse, and several cases of pseudo-Bartter's syndrome have appeared in the literature.[18,205,394,436]

Also of consideration are idiopathic, cyclical, and periodic edema.[13,81,94,412] These problems have been the subject of considerable discussion in the medical literature. They are most often manifest in women who have problems with excess fluid retention—usually premenstrual, but the edema can be independent of the menstrual cycle.[412] Women with idiopathic edema are at times prescribed diuretics for the problem, and several studies suggest that idiopathic edema may not really be idiopathic, but may instead be linked to the misuse of diuretics, although clearly this is not true in all cases.[281,282,445]

It is important to remember that people may obtain diuretics in several ways: (1) over-the-counter, (2) for appropriate or questionably appropriate medical conditions, (3) by seeking prescriptions from multiple physicians who are unaware that the drug is being prescribed by others, (4) by using someone else's diuretics (a not uncommon problem among women with bulimia nervosa), and (5) by stealing diuretics in the work place. A

Table 11. Commonly Available Over-the-Counter Diet Pills[a]

Brand	Amounts	Recommended[b] Dosage/Day
Acutrim® 16 Hour	75 mg	1
Acutrim II® Max. Duration	75 mg	1
Appendrine® Max. Strength	25 mg	3
Control® Max. Strength	75 mg	1
Dexatrim®	50 mg	1
Dexatrim® Extra Strength[c]	75 mg	1
Dexatrim® 15	75 mg	1
Dietac®	75 mg	1
Prolamine™ Max. Strength®	37.5 mg	2
Super Odrinex®	25 mg	3

[a]Active appetite suppressor in all brands is phenylpropanolamine HCL; several brands also contain vitamins, minerals, and iron.
[b]Recommended package dosing schedule.
[c]Two formulations available: Extra Strength with Vit. C and Caffeine-Free Extra Strength.

number of cases of diuretic abuse have occurred in health care personnel who had access to diuretics.

The three groups of prescription diuretics most commonly used for control of idiopathic edema or premenstrual edema, and most often abused with patients with eating disorders, are the thiazides, the loop diuretics, and the potassium-sparing diuretics.[23] Adverse consequences of the thiazide diuretics include hypokalemia, cardiac conduction defects, arrhythmias, hypokalemic nephropathy, and cardiomyopathy.[23,384,419] Loop diuretics include furosemide and ethacrynic acid. The most common problems with these drugs are orthostatic hypotension and hypokalemic metabolic alkalosis; hyperuricemia, hypocalcemia, ototoxicity, and magnesium depletion can also occur.[23] Potassium-sparing diuretics, including spironolactone and triameterene, usually result in mild hyperkalemic acidosis, and trameterene can result in nephrolithiasis and acute renal failure.[23]

In our experience, most patients with bulimia ingest over-the-counter diuretics.[310] These are summarized in table 12. It is hard to evaluate the risks of these medications. Most contain Pamabron, ammonium chloride, and/or caffeine. The effects of these over-the-counter diuretics in individuals with eating disorders, many of whom have other abnormalities owing to vomiting and laxative abuse, are unknown.

Table 12. Commonly Available Over-the-Counter Diuretics[a]

Brand	Active Diuretic Ingredients	Amount	Recommended Dosage/Day
Premesyn-PMS®	Pamabrom (with 15 mg pyrilamine maleate)	25 mg	8/day
Sunril®Premenstrual Capsules	Pamabrom (with 25 mg pyrilamine maleate)	50 mg	4/day
Midol-PMS®	Pamabrom (with 15 mg pyrilamine maleate)	25 mg	8/day
Odrinil®	Pamabrom	25 mg	8/day
Diurex-MPR®	Pamabrom	25 mg	8/day (no more than 10 consecutive days/month except by M.D. recommendation)
Pamprin Menstrual Relief®	Pamabrom (with 15 mg pyrilamine maleate)	25 mg	8/day
Aqua-Ban®	Ammonium chloride Caffeine	325 mg 100 mg	6/day (no more than 6 days/month)
Maximum Strength Aqua-Ban Plus®	Ammonium chloride Caffeine	650 mg 200 mg	3/day (no more than 6 days/month)
Odrinil™ Natural Diruetic®	Caffeine (with herbal extracts)	Not specified	4/day
Diurex®	Caffeine (with uva ursi, buchu)	Not specified	4/day

[a]Preparations containing only a small amount of caffeine and therefore having limited diuretic effects are not included in this table.

Ipecac

Ipecac syrup is dispensed in the United States in bottles containing 30 cc of the syrup, equivalent to 21 mg of emetine base. The ipecac alkaloid emetine is responsible for the development of myopathies, including cardiomyopathies,[5,40,115,285,319,346] if the drug is ingested repeatedly over a short period of time.

The only prevalence data concerning ipecac and eating disorders were published by Pope and colleagues in 1986.[363] They found that of 100 consecutive patients presenting for treatment, 28 had reported using ipecac, and of these, 3 had abused the drug at least 100 times, and one patient had ingested the drug more than 2,000 times. Medical management of patients who use ipecac includes assessment for possible complications and discontinuation of the drug. The major concerns are cardiomyopathy and peripheral myopathy. Careful assessment of cardiovascular status, including electrocardiogram and ecocardiography, should be undertaken.

It needs to be stressed that when asking patients about ipecac usage, one should also educate them about the risks of the drug, so as not to inadvertently suggest use of the drug. The ingestion of nicotine to stimulate vomiting has also been reported.[407]

Medical Evaluation

There are several general screening procedures and tests that are indicated for all patients who present with bulimia nervosa, and several specific procedures and tests that are indicated in certain situations. However, it must be stressed that with all patients, a careful history, directed to uncovering problem behaviors that might cause serious medical complications, is the most important source of information for which no laboratory tests can substitute. Such problems as laxative abuse, diuretic abuse, and the use of ipecac must be asked routinely. A direct, forthright, nonjudgmental approach is best. Second, all patients need a careful physical examination, with careful attention to evidence of dehydration or GI bleeding.

Serum electrolytes should be checked routinely in all patients. The prevalence of fluid and electrolyte abnormalities, at times severe, is so high that it would be negligent not to evaluate electrolyte function prior to treatment.

Beyond electrolyte determinations, the specific items of the history, the complaints of the patient, and the findings on physical examination should direct the physician to the necessity for further evaluation. A number of tests are highly desirable for the screening of these patients, and others can be reserved for specific situations. these are summarized in table 13.

I cannot overemphasize that medical screening and evaluation should be considered a necessary part of the evaluation and treatment of all patients with bulimia nervosa. Nonphysician therapists who work with these

Table 13. Suggested Evaluation Procedures for Patients with Bulmia Nervosa

Essential:	1. Complete history
	2. Complete physical examination
	3. Serum electrolytyes (Na, K, Cl, HCO_3)
	4. Stool exam for blood
Strongly Recommended:	1. CBC
	2. Serum BUN, creatinine, glucose
	3. Serum cal., phos.
	4. Screening liver function tests
	5. EKG
	6. T3, T4
	7. Serum amylase
	8. Dental examination
Consider:	1. CT of head (or MRI)
	2. EEG
	3. Electromyography
	4. Urine screen for diuretics/laxatives
	5. GI radiographic/scoping procedures if evidence of GI blood loss

patients need to develop a close relationship with a physician who can supervise this element of the evaluation. Put simply, therapists who are unwilling to take the responsibility to see that the necessary medical evaluation and monitoring are accomplished should not be involved in the care of these patients, and should instead refer them to someone who is willing to assume such a role.

6

Psychobiology of Bulimia Nervosa

Over the last few decades knowledge in the field of neurobiology, has dramatically increased, and it is safe to say that advances in this area are among the most important and innovative in all of science. A part of this increase in knowledge has been a marked expansion of our understanding of the biological mechanisms that regulate weight, appetite, and feeding. Although much of this research has yet to be translated into human applications, attempts are now being made to bridge the basic science and the clinical—to use basic science findings to generate theories about the causes of eating problems and to develop novel treatment strategies for patients with eating disorders, including bulimia nervosa.[322,323]

As part of our discussion, it is important to review some of the basic mechanisms involved in the control of feeding behavior. This review will better prepare us to examine several of the studies in which researchers have applied these findings to clinical populations. We will start with the basic control systems that have received the most attention—the catecholamine neurotransmitter norepinephrine, the indoleamine neurotransmitter serotonin, and the peptide neurotransmitters/neuromodulators, all of which appear to be active in the area of the brain that controls eating—the hypothalamus.[266]

Neurotransmitters/Neuromodulators

Studies in animals have shown that the catecholamine neurotransmitter norepinephrine (NE) stimulates feeding in animals when released into the hypothalamus, even if the animals have been satiated through previous food exposure.[266] NE release appears to engender a preferential increase in carbohydrate intake. This observation has been used to explain why antidepressant drugs may cause some depressed patients to crave carbohydrates and to gain weight, presumably owing to their inhibition of the reuptake inactivation of norepinephrine, which makes more NE available in the synapse.

Traditionally, clinical investigators have focused on the evaluation of neurotransmitters in anorexia nervosa.[3,131,141,147,149] However, recently, investigators have used various approaches to evaluate neurotransmitter function, including norepinephrine function, in patients with normal-weight bulimia.

Pirke and colleagues reported that patients with bulimia nervosa had blunted plasma norepinephrine responses to standing, suggesting dysfunction in the NE system.[354] Jimmerson, Kaye, and their colleagues have reported studies using pharmacological challenge tests with isoprotorenol, an adrenergic agonist, to examine NE functioning indirectly.[207] Isoprotorenol was used to evaluate beta adrenoreceptor sensitivity in bulimic patients who had been stabilized nutritionally and metabolically. The hypothesis guiding this approach is that beta adrenoreceptor function may be up-regulated, or overly sensitive, in bulimia nervosa patients. This hypothesis follows from the observations that many bulimic patients improve on antidepressants, and that antidepressants have been shown to down-regulate postsynaptic receptor activity and/or decrease presynaptic release. Also these authors were interested in evaluating the possible role of beta adrenoreceptor function in the metabolic rate disturbance seen in these patients. If altered sensitivity of the beta adrenoreceptor were to be found, as demonstrated by a reduced lipolytic response to isoprotorenol administration, this might help to explain the reduced caloric requirements necessary for weight maintenance that has been demonstrated in individuals with bulimia nervosa.

All subjects tested were free of medication and hospitalized on the research unit at the National Institute of Mental Health. Control subjects were matched for age and body weight. The results indicated that baseline levels of free fatty acid and isoproterenol-induced release were quite similar between patients and controls. However, the bulimic patients had a significantly reduced mean resting pulse and mean systolic blood pressure and, consistent with this finding, lower mean plasma norepinephrine levels. The authors also found an increased chronotropic effect for isoproterenol. This was interpreted as showing up-regulation of the cardiovascular beta adrenoreceptors, which might develop to compensate for a lower presynaptic release of norepinephrine. The pathophysiology of the reduction of plasma norepinephrine is unclear, although the authors speculated that it might relate to the restricted caloric intake practiced by many of these patients. This group has also demonstrated increased responsiveness of B-adrenergic receptors in circulating lymphocytes in bulimics compared to controls.[41]

The authors also found increased anxiety ratings during the infusion of isoproterenol in patients compared to controls. In attempting to synthesize their results with clinical knowledge about these disorders, these authors speculated that high levels of anxiety might be associated with the precipitation of binge-eating episodes. Binge-eating results in an increase in circulating norepinephrine, which would induce a down-regulation of peripheral adrenoreceptors and result in a transient decrease in anxiety. This finding might explain the decrease in anxiety reported by bulimic patients after binge-eating and vomiting.

Another neurotransmitter, serotonin, usually produces effects opposite to those of norepinephrine on food intake, causing a reduction, in particular a preferential reduction in carbohydrate intake, in animals.[266] There are potential correlates in humans for this observation. Cyproheptadine, a serotonin antagonist, tends to stimulate weight gain in humans.[22,133,333,411,453] Cyproheptadine also facilitates appetite and improves the rate of weight gain in restrictor anorectics, while not benefiting, and in some cases actually worsening, the bulimic symptoms in bulimic anorectics.[150,151] Fenfluramine, a drug that facilitates serotonergic transmission, has been shown to suppress craving for carbohydrates in humans. These observations suggest the possibility of inadequate serotonin input into hypothalamic regulator mechanisms in bulimic patients.

Other research has demonstrated that the administration of serotonin precursors or serotonin agonists will reduce food consumption, particularly the consumption of carbohydrate-rich food, with a relative sparing of protein intake. Wurtman and Wurtman have conducted a considerable amount of research into the regulation of carbohydrate intake, focusing on the hypothesis that carbohydrate intake is regulated separately from overall caloric intake.[481,482] They have studied subjects who reported that they had a tendency to snack on high-carbohydrate foods. The administration of the drug fenfluramine, significantly decreased the carbohydrate snack intake in these individuals.

These authors further investigated the possibility that there was an abnormality in serotonin regulation of carbohydrate intake in studies using obese human subjects. In a closely monitored inpatient setting obese subjects consumed very few protein snacks but large amounts of carbohydrate snacks. The administration of fenfluramine suppressed carbohydrate eating during snacks and, in a subsequent study, during regular meals as well. These authors concluded that a subgroup of obese individuals, so-called carbohydrate cravers, consume excessive amounts of carbohydrate-rich foods, and that this pattern may result from abnormal regulation of the neurotransmitter serotonin. They have further hypothesized that the increased carbohydrate intake might represent an attempt on the part of these individuals to enhance serotonin transmission centrally, which theoretically might result in mood elevation.

The synthesis of brain serotonin is enhanced by eating calorie-rich, low-protein foods, while eating high protein foods inhibits serotonin synthesis. Many of the amino acids in high-protein foods compete with tryptophan, the precursor of serotonin, for uptake into the brain; therefore, if these amino acids are ingested, they may reduce the amount of tryptophan that can get into the brain and be available for serotonin synthesis. To further evaluate the possibility that carbohydrate intake was driven by this mechanism, "carbohydrate cravers" were given high-carbohydrate meals and their mood changes were compared to those of a comparison group of obese subjects whose eating patterns were not characterized by high-carbohydrate snack foods. Carbohydrate cravers experienced more of an improvement in mood than did the controls, supporting the hypothesis.

Analogous to this line of reasoning, bulimic behavior can be conceptualized as the result of hypofunctioning of serotonergic systems. This hypothesis is compatible with several other observations: (1) A high prevalence of depression occurs in patients with bulimia nervosa. Response to antidepressant drugs has often been linked to their effects on biogenic amines, including serotonin, the presumption being that serotonin function is low in depressed individuals, and that transmission in the system is enhanced by antidepressants at least on a short-term basis. (2) Low levels of serotonin metabolites have been described in some patients with depression, particularly in the subgroup characterized by impulsivity.[36]

Based on such observations, it is reasonable to investigate serotonin function in bulimic patients.

As recently summarized by Jimerson, Kaye, Brewerton, and their colleagues, there are several ways of assessing serotonin activity.[37,206] One is to measure the metabolite 5-hydroxy-indoleacetic acid (5-HIAA) in cerebrospinal fluid (CSF). Studies of CSF 5-HIAA have not, to my knowledge, been reported for patients of normal weight with bulimia nervosa. However, such studies have been done for patients with anorexia nervosa. Kaye and colleagues have found that the CSF 5-HIAA levels, measured following the administration of probenicide—a drug that causes the accumulation of 5-HIAA in CSF—are higher in nonbulimics than in bulimic subgroups.[233] This suggests that the nonbulimic anorectics may have increased brain serotonin metabolism relative to the bulimic subgroup, which suggests a deficiency or hypofunctioning in the subgroup characterized by bulimic symptoms. This same group of investigators has also demonstrated a blunted prolactin response to the administration of the serotonin precursor L-tryptophan and to the oral administration of the serotonin postsynaptic receptor agonist m-chlorophenylpiperazine (M-CPP), again suggesting the possibility of hypofunctioning of serotonin in bulimics.[207]

Kaye and colleagues have also examined the hypothesis,[234] mentioned previously, that binge-eating may represent on attempt to elevate plasma and brain tryptophan levels and to enhance brain serotonin. They have compared the levels of tryptophan in serum to the serum levels of the large neutral amino acids, which compete with tryptophan for the same uptake sites into the brain (tryptophan/LNAA ratio). During binge-eating and vomiting episodes those bulimic subjects who exhibit an increase in the TRP/LNAA ratio are the ones who self-terminate binge-eating, while those who do not demonstrate this elevation tend to continue to binge-eat and vomit. These data suggest that one possible biological signal for the termination of binge-eating behavior is the elevation of the TRP/LNAA ratio, which may correlate with increased serotonin availability in the brain and, theoretically, improvement in mood. These data support the possibility of hyposerotonergic functioning in some patients with bulimia nervosa and suggest that binge-eating represents an attempt to compensate for this deficit.

Peptidergic (protein) neurotransmitters also are important in the regulation of appetite and weight, and several peptidergic systems have been investigated.[321, 325] We will focus on two that have been of particular interest in the regulation of feeding. One system uses the peptide neurotransmitter cholecystokinin (CCK).[416,417] Early in the 1970s cholecystokinin was shown to cause a dose-related decrease in food intake when administrated parenterally in rats. CCK has activity in many animal models. In some species, e.g., the rat, CCK appears to act peripherally through binding to receptors in the vagal system, since vagotomy will abolish the effect. However, in other species, such as the dog, an intact vagal system is not necessary for the effect of the drug, which appears to be working through a separate mechanism.

Cholecystokinin octapeptide (CCK-8), the molecular form of the peptide that has been synthesized, has been administered experimentally to humans to evaluate its satiety effects. Although initial studies using an impure form of CCK were negative, subsequent reports using the synthesized peptide have, for the most part, suggested a satiety affect, particularly when the drug was administered by constant infusion during eating.[138,355,405,427] The effect does not appear to be secondary to nausea.

Our group administered CCK intravenously to bulimia nervosa patients hospitalized on a metabolic research ward in order to see if augmentation of CCK would terminate binge-eating. The results demonstrated no difference between placebo and active CCK-8 administration.[306] However, only one dosage was used, and it is certainly possible that at a different dosage the peptide might have a significant effect. Geracioti and Liddle recently published that bulimic patients had imparied CCK reaction in response to a test meal, suggesting that CCK might be deficient in these patients and may contribute to their impaired satiety.[128]

Another family of peptides that has been extensively evaluated for its involvement in feeding is the opioid peptide system.[322] Beginning with studies in the early 1970s, it was demonstrated that the analgesic effect of opioids was mediated through stereospecific interactions with opiate receptors in the central nervous system. Subsequently substances with opiate-like effects were isolated and purified. Eventually several groups of opioid peptides were discovered, and their importance was found to extend far beyond their role in pain modulation, to include various other physiological processes such as feeding.

Martin and colleagues first reported that opiate agonists stimulated feeding, and that morphine-dependent rats would overfeed following administration of the drug.[287] Lowy demonstrated that this hyperphagia was reversible using the short-acting narcotic (opiate) antagonist naloxone.[279] Holtzman in 1974 demonstrated that naloxone would decrease feeding in rats who had not received exogenous opiates following food deprivation.[175] This observation was later confirmed in various reports across several different species involving different feeding paradigms, including tail-pinch-induced feeding, diazepam-induced eating, and feeding induced by the administration of the glucose antimetabolite 2-Deoxyglucose.[307] The feeding suppression was shown to be dose dependent and stereospecific, and not mediated by taste aversion. Tail-pinch-induced feeding, one model for studying feeding in rats, is thought to represent a possible animal model of stress-induced eating. Feeding using the model was also antagonized by narcotic antagonists, suggesting that stress-induced overeating in humans might be responsive to opiate antagonists.[324]

Because of these observations, several researchers have administered opiate antagonists to humans in an attempt to suppress feeding. There have been both case reports and reports of series of obese individuals who were given naloxone, as well as anecdotal reports concerning the long-acting narcotic antagonist naltrexone, all suggesting that the drug may have an appetite-suppressant effect. We will briefly review these reports.

Hollister in 1981 reported decreased food intake in 6 of 10 nonaddict normals taking naltrexone,[174] and Sternbach in 1982 observed anorectic effects in detoxified opiate addicts.[421] Several investigators then demonstrated experimentally that the short-term administration of naloxone would reduce feeding in obese humans and, in some work, normal-weight humans. The effect apparently was not secondary to an alteration in the perception of satiety or fullness. Because of these observations, systematically controlled studies of the long-acting narcotic antagonist naltrexone were conducted in humans with obesity.[12,283,284,307,308] Various dosages of naltrexone, ranging from 50 to 300 mg per day, were employed. With the exception of one study (in which a secondary analysis by sex indicated that women taking the active drug lost slightly but significantly more weight compared to women on placebo), all of these reports have been negative. However, our group and others have recently turned their attention to the possibility that narcotic antagonists may be useful in the treatment of bulimia nervosa. In one short-term administration study, we demonstrated that naloxone infusion attenuated binge-eating behavior in hospitalized bulimic subjects, and Jonas and Gold, in an ongoing open-label study using naltrexone, found considerable benefit for this drug. These results are reviewed in the chapter on psychopharmacology.

Several groups of investigators have recently started to measure peptides involved in the control of feeding in the CSF and plasma of patients with bulimia nervosa. Fullerton and colleagues have found elevations of plasma beta endorphin in patients with bulimia nervosa, but the elevation was found only in patients who were actively vomiting, suggesting that the elevation resulted from rather than caused the bulimic symptoms.[117,118] Waller and colleagues found evidence of decreased beta endorphin in the plasma of bulimics.[455] Kaye and colleagues have reported elevation of somatostatin levels in the CSF of bulimics,[235] and elevations in CSF peptide YY after 1 month of abstinence (personal communication). This later finding is particularly interesting, as PYY is a very potent feeding stimulator in various species.

Neuroendocrine Functioning

Neuroendocrine functioning has been evaluated in patients with eating disorders for several reasons: 1) It was hoped that studying these systems would help in delineating and understanding the physiological sequelae of eating disorders, 2) Neuroendocrine abnormalities are commonly seen in patients with other types of psychiatric disorders, and such abnormalities have been of particular interest in studies of affective disorders. The high prevalence of affective symptoms in many bulimia patients suggests that some cases of bulimia nervosa may represent variants of affective disorder; a search for types of neuroendocrine dysfunctions that may be common in both disorders has been pursued. 3) Neuroendocrine regulatory systems are centered in the hypothalamus, an area of the brain of particular interest to those who study the psychobiology of eating and weight.

Adrenal activity has been investigated intensively in patients with anorexia nervosa, and these studies indicate that anorectic patients generally have elevated plasma cortisol levels, owing both to slow metabolism of cortisol and an excess production of cortisol. Such changes are also seen in individuals who are malnourished for other reasons.

As mentioned previously there has also been considerable interest in hypothalamic/pituitary/adrenal control mechanisms in depression.[51,52] Of particular interest have been the lack of adrenal suppression using the dexamethasone-suppression test (DST), the loss of the normal diurnal variation in cortisol secretion, and hyperfunctioning of the entire axis in many depressed patients.

Several groups of investigators have also studied dexamethansone suppression in patients with bulimia nervosa.[145,183,197,228,244,274,276,316,327, 340,347] The usual methodology has been to administer 1 mg of dexamethasone at 11 p.m. and obtain plasma cortisol levels the following day at 4 p.m. and/or 11 p.m. Postdexamethasone plasma levels of cortisol are usually considered normal if they are less than 5 mcg/deciliter. Several of the studies examining DST in normal-weight bulimia are summarized in table 14. The majority of these studies found rates of nonsuppression much higher than those seen in studies of normals and, in several of the studies, compared to age-matched controls. However, there has not been a consistent association between nonsuppression and concomitant affective symptoms or weight loss, and the reason for the elevated rate of DST nonsuppression was not elucidated in these early studies.[91]

However, Walsh and colleagues recently reported the results of a study in which they sampled cortisol repeatedly over a 24-hour period. The results indicated that the cortisol levels in bulimic patients were similar to those of normal controls, suggesting normal hypothalamo-pituitary-adrenal axis (HPA) activity. Walsh and colleagues also demonstrated a probable explanation for the lack of suppression on the DST, by showing that although plasma levels of dexamethasone varied a great deal among bulimic patients, mean plasma levels of dexamethasone were significantly lower than in the controls.[457] Also, there was a highly significant negative correlation between plasma levels of cortisol and plasma levels of dexamethasone, suggesting that the low levels of plasma dexamethasone may account for the high rate of lack of suppression of cortisol on the DST. Therefore, DST nonsuppression may be an effect of poor absorption of the dexamethasone, perhaps owing to the problem of loss of dexamethasone through vomiting, or through some other mechanism that impairs absorption.

Metabolic changes have also been reported in association with bulimia nervosa. Pirke and associates found that patients with bulimia nervosa tended to have lower serum glucose levels, reduced T3 levels, reduced plasma norepinephrine response to postural change, and elevated levels of free fatty acid and beta hydroxybutyric acid, a metabolic pattern suggestive of dietary deficiencies, despite a normal weight in these patients.[352]

Table 14. Dexamethasone-Suppression Test in Bulimia

Author(s)	Year	N	Samples	Rate of Nonsuppression
Hudson et al.	1982	9	4 pm	56%
Gwirtsman et al.	1983	18	4 pm, 11 pm	67%
Hudson et al.	1983	47	4 pm	47%
Mitchell et al.	1984	28	4 pm, 11 pm	50%
Lindy et al.	1985	55	4 pm	35%
Musisi et al.	1985	20	4 pm	20%
Kiriike et al.	1986	8	4 pm	63%
Hughes et al.	1986	23	4 pm, 11 pm	48%
Levy et al.	1987	8	4 pm, 10 pm	100%
Perez et al.	1988	33	4 pm	58%
O'Brien et al.	1988	19	4 pm	47%

Several researchers have examined the relationship between bulimia nervosa and plasma glucose regulation. Ferguson reported a bulimic individual who died suddenly and whose death was attributed to acute hypoglycemia.[108] Two subsequent studies found no significant abnormalities with glucose tolerance in patients with bulimia, while one study, which used an adequate control group, found glucose regulation abnormalities in this population.[173,293,464] Further work is indicated in this area.

Patients with bulimia nervosa frequently have irregular menses; however, only a minority develop the profound amenorrhea seen in anorexia nervosa. Several explanations have been offered for these menstrual abnormalities, including the weight fluctuations seen in these patients, the starvation effects of the eating disorder, and the excessive exercise pattern some of these patients practice. Pirke and colleagues have studied hypothalamic-pituitary-ovarian function in patients with bulimia nervosa.[350,351] In their study, 6 of 30 patients had amenorrhea or oligomenorrhea. Prolactin values were not elevated in the bulimic individuals compared to controls, suggesting that hyperprolactinemia is an unlikely cause for the menstrual cycle dysfunction. However, they found that 12-hour FSH levels were significantly lower in the bulimic patients than in the controls, and hypothesized that this might be responsible for impaired estradiol secretion. They also found reduced peak levels of LH and FSH in some bulimic patients; however, the frequencies of FSH and LH peaks were unaltered.

Seven studies, including a total of 83 subjects, have examined TRH-

Table 15. TSH Response to TRH in Bulimia

Author(s)	Year	N	Rate of Blunting	Rate of Delayed Peak
Gwirtsman et al.	1983	10	80%	20%
Mitchell et al.	1983	6	17%	0%
Norris et al.	1985	10	30%	30%
Levy et al.	1986	7	14%	57%
Kaplan et al.	1986	19	0%	0%
Kiriike	1987	9	0%	22%
Kiyohara et al.	1988	8	13%	38%

Table 16. Abnormal GH Response to TRH in Bulimia

Author(s)	Year	N	Rate of Abnormal Increase
Gwirtsman et al.	1983	3	67%
Mitchell et al.	1983	6	67%
Kiriike et al.	1987	9	11%

induced TSH releases in bulimia nervosa (table 15).[145,228,244,247,274,293,339] Of the patients studied, 20% had a blunted TSH response to TRH. However, in all of these studies less than one third of the subjects demonstrated this abnormality (with the exception of the study by Gwirtsman and colleagues in which a higher rate was found). Therefore the exact rate of blunting is apparently low and its significance unclear.

A few authors have also reported abnormal GH response to TRH in bulimia, but the number of subjects studied has been quite small and the significance of this abnormality is unknown (Table 16).

Sleep Architecture

There is a large body of literature indicating that a subgroup of patients with major depressive disorder have certain demonstrable abnormalities on sleep EEG, including shortened REM latency. Several groups of investigators have studied sleep parameters in patients with bulimia nervosa, again to delineate possible similarities between depression and this disorder. Weilberg and colleagues[469] in 1985 reported that patients with bulimia had long REM latencies, but noted "REM-like periods" earlier than expected for REM onset. However, subsequent reports by Walsh and colleagues,[461] Levy and colleagues,[275] and Hudson and colleagues,[190] involving a total of 35 patients with bulimia nervosa failed to demonstrate any consistent changes in sleep EEG that were different from the patterns of normal control women. In particular, the sorts of changes seen in major depression were not found.

7

Nutritional Counseling

Many mental health professionals who work with bulimia patients have a very limited background in nutritional science. Also of interest, the dieticians who work with these patients generally have a rather limited training in counseling techniques. Both of these limitations are unfortunate, in that both psychotherapy and nutritional counseling are important in the treatment of this disorder. Integration of these treatment aspects can be accomplished in several ways. Many programs use a team approach, wherein a dietician is responsible for the nutritional counseling elements and someone else is responsible for the psychotherapy and/or pharmacotherapy components. However, such an arrangement is impractical in many settings, where the services of a dietician are not readily available. Therefore, it is highly desirable for mental health practitioners who work with eating disorders to have a solid working knowledge in nutrition, since it is of utmost importance that nutritional counseling be implemented early as a component in the treatment of these disorders.

In this chapter I will discuss some of the nutritional information that therapists should possess, and that they should teach their patients, and outline a simple meal-planning system that can be taught early in therapy.

I. Self-Assessment. A good way to introduce the discussion of nutritional issues is to have patients record everything they eat, binge-foods and otherwise, for at least a 24-hour period, and to carefully review that record during the next session. The patterns of food intake—whether or not they are eating regular meals, whether the meals are adequately balanced, the nature of the relationship between binge-eating and fasting—all should be addressed.

II. Roles of Food and Eating. It is important for patients to understand what roles food and eating have in their lives. Possible roles include the following:

A. Sustenance. Food supplies the biological sustenance necessary for human physiology. Many bulimic women take inadequate amounts of some nutrients and are "starved" even at a normal weight.

B. Socialization. Many social gatherings involve food, and many people like to go out to eat with others. This is very problematic for women with bulimia nervosa, who tend to binge-eat in private and feel very self-conscious about eating with others. The impact of this pattern on social relationships should be reviewed.

C. Pleasure. Many people eat food because it is pleasurable. Certain foods, such as desserts and snack foods, are particularly enjoyable for many people. Many people use pleasurable foods for rewards, such as eating a candy bar after studying. Many women with bulimia nervosa have difficulty enjoying food unless they are binge-eating and planning to vomit. Rather than being pleasureful, food becomes "the enemy."

D. Comfort. Many people use food to comfort themselves; likewise many individuals with bulimia nervosa use binge-eating to comfort themselves when they are anxious, depressed, or upset about something.

E. Distraction. Many people with eating problems such as bulimia nervosa use food to distract themselves from unpleasant tasks or affects; food becomes a way to "put off" other things.

F. Guilt and Shame. For many individuals with bulimia nervosa, eating becomes a source of guilt and shame. They feel they should not eat at all unless they are binge-eating, and binge-eating in itself leads to depression and shame.

As part of this discussion, have the patient make a list of the roles that food and eating have in her life, and review this list in therapy.

III. Monitoring Eating Behavior. To better understand the role of food and eating in her life, it is important for the patient to keep further records of her eating behavior for several days, and to begin to link these eating behaviors to specific thoughts or feelings. These thoughts or feelings may occur before, during, or after the eating behavior. A sample form is

For Day:			Name:	
FOOD ITEM		AMOUNT	THOUGHTS Linked with eating	FEELINGS Linked with eating
TIME				
TIME				
TIME				

Figure 3. Daily Eating Log

shown as figure 3. It is important to stress to the patient that she list *every-thing* that she eats.

Carefully review these records. In particular, notice specific thoughts or feelings that recur in relationship to eating. Particularly common among individuals with bulimia nervosa are binge-eating in response to anxiety or depression, feeling out of control while eating, feeling afraid after eating, and feeling depressed and guilty after vomiting.

IV. Education About Nutrition. Review with patients the importance of foods and nutrients in providing energy, in fueling the body processes, and in growth and maintenance of body tissues. While many different systems can be used, I generally teach patients to think in terms of six groups of nutrients: carbohydrates, proteins, fats, vitamins, minerals, and water. The first three of these provide energy directly and will be discussed later.

Vitamins are primarily involved in the regulation of body processes, which include absorption of nutrients from the digestive tract, energy-producing reactions in cells, and protein building.

Minerals are involved in building healthy tissues, such as bones and teeth, and are important in the regulation of muscle contraction and nerve conduction. Calcium is of particular importance for patients with problem eating behaviors, since they are apparently at increased risk for osteoporosis. Several factors may contribute to the development of osteoporosis, including low estrogen levels, low calcium intake—quite common in these patients—and too little exercise. Also, it is common for patients with bulimia nervosa to eliminate dairy products from their diet. Stress that women who are menstruating should consume the equivalent of two to four cups of milk or yogurt each day. Women who are not menstruating regularly probably require more. For individuals who cannot tolerate milk, yogurt, cheese, salmon, sardines with bones, or oysters are reasonable alternatives.

Water is considered a separate nutrient in this system, because water intake is a problem for many patients with eating disorders, who may be dehydrated from vomiting, laxative or diuretic abuse, or excessive exercise. It is important to encourage patients to take in six to eight cups of water daily and to try to limit caffeine-containing fluids, since such beverages do not improve hydration status because of their diuretic effects.

We turn now to the energy nutrients. In discussing energy nutrients it is important to understand each patient's perceptions, and often misperceptions, about these nutrients. First, ask the patient what foods come to mind when you mention carbohydrates, fats, and proteins. Second, have the patient "evaluate" these foods. Do they see these foods as healthy, unhealthy, neutral, forbidden? What tends to make each of these foods healthy or unhealthy? Forbidden?

For many patients with eating disorders, carbohydrates are regarded as good or bad depending on the type of carbohydrate. Carbohydrates in fruits and vegetables are often considered healthy, while carbohydrates in sugar, refined flour, desserts, and candies are considered unhealthy and forbidden, unless one intends to vomit. As in many other areas of life, individuals with bulimia nervosa get into all-or-nothing thinking about such foods. When a bulimic is eating in a "healthy" way, she should not eat refined carbohydrates or high-fat foods, since one bite may trigger a binge-eating episode. However, when binge-eating, high-fat, high-carbohydrate foods are often preferred.

It is important to encourage patients to try to broaden their list of approved foods, and to point out that both "good and bad" foods are permissible, if one is familiar with their nutrient content and if one balances each food with others to make sure that the overall nutrient intake represents the proper amount of each energy nutrient.

Stress to patients that carbohydrates are the preferred form of fuel for the human body and that certain tissues, particularly the brain and other nervous tissue, rely almost exclusively on carbohydrates for fuel. General recommendations are that at least 50% of the energy intake should be from carbohydrates.

As with carbohydrates, it is important to discuss protein. When asked what foods come to mind, many people answer fish, poultry, cheese, and milk.

However, it is important to point out to patients that legumes, breads, cereals, vegetables, peanut butter, nuts, and seeds are also high in protein. Do they see protein as healthy or unhealthy? Most patients with eating disorders indicate that red meat, such as beef or lamb, is unhealthy. While it is known that many adults should limit their intake of red meat in order to decrease their cholesterol and saturated fat intake, most patients with bulimia nervosa take this to the extreme. "Reduce red meat" gets translated into "cut out all red meat" or "all red meat is bad." Indeed, red meat provides an excellent source of high-quality protein and iron, and a moderate intake of red meat should be encouraged.

Point out that protein is essential for building and repairing tissues, and that protein cannot be stored in the body like fats and carbohydrates. Protein should make up 12 to 20% of the nutrient intake.

We then turn to that most detestable nutrient, fat. For many patients with eating disorders, the first thing that comes to mind when they hear the word fat is body fat; food fat = body fat. The belief is that eating foods that contain fat, such as butter, margarine, or chocolate, translates into fat on the abdominal wall, hips, or thighs. This, of course, is a misconception. Any energy nutrient — carbohydrate, protein, or fat — eaten in excess eventually results in excess body fat, and any energy nutrient, including fat eaten in moderation, will be burned as fuel.

Because the word *fat* is so clearly linked with body fat, in our program we refer to it as the satiety nutrient, emphasizing its role in providing a sense of satiety or satisfaction after eating. This nutrient is found in most meat, fish, and poultry, as well as butter, margarine, and salad dressing. it is also commonly present in bakery items, dairy products, and in many casseroles. Stress that patients should get some satiety nutrient with each meal.

V. Food Deprivation. Patients need to appreciate the relationship between the food deprivation that they experience when not binge-eating and their subsequent binge-eating behavior. The usual pattern for bulimia nervosa patients is to attempt to eat as little as possible when not binge-eating. This state of relative food deprivation leads to obsessive thoughts about food, poor concentration, irritability, and mood lability; then binge-eating breaks through. The fear engendered by the binge-eating then leads to vomiting and/or laxative abuse, and to a strong resolve to skip meals, again as a way of preventing weight gain or promoting weight loss. Therefore, bulimia nervosa is a disorder not just of binge-eating and vomiting, but of binge-eating and food deprivation. Most patients with bulimia nervosa eat quite poorly most of the time. Therefore, it is important for the patient to understand that the goal of treatment is not just to eliminate the binge-eating and other associated bulimic behaviors such as vomiting, but also to institute a plan of eating regular balanced meals.

Most patients are initially quite resistant to this suggestion. Many are convinced that if they start to eat regular balanced meals, they will gain weight. It is important for the therapist to assume a nonjudgmental but firm position — it is of utmost importance for the patient to start eating regular balanced meals and to plan those meals in advance.

I think advance meal planning has a number of advantages. First, it allows the patient to retrain herself as to how she should be eating. She should be explicitly told not to eat because she is hungry, not to quit when she is full, and not to respond to external cues, but instead initially to follow the meal plan—to eat what she should be eating, when she should be eating it. Most will try to "cut corners" and omit certain foods. Again, they should be strongly encouraged to follow the meal plan as closely as possible.

VI. Meal Planning. The goal of this system is to teach the patients to eat three balanced meals a day with or without snacks. They should be instructed to try to eat these meals at fairly standard times when possible. One way to approach the planning is to separate foods into six basic food groups, including:

Primary proteins—meats, fish, poultry, cheese, legumes, eggplant
Satiety foods—butter, margarine, oil, salad dressing
Grains and energy-rich vegetables—bread, cereals, crackers, potatoes, corn, green peas
Vegetables—string beans, tomatoes, carrots
Fruits—fruit, fruit juice, sugar
Calcium-rich foods—milk, yogurt, ice cream
Fluids—water, caffeine-free beverages

Point out to the patient that the energy-rich vegetables are so named because they have almost three times the amount of carbohydrates as other vegetables, with the same relative amount of protein.

This system uses the term "food unit" as a basic unit of measure and attempts to get patients away from counting calories. For example, a fruit unit is a basic unit of measurement within the fruit group. One-half of a large banana and one medium orange are both equivalent to one fruit unit, because they have the same approximate proportion of energy nutrients and are therefore interchangeable. However, one unit is not always one portion. For example, one ounce of turkey is equivalent to one primary protein unit, but an average portion of turkey would be two to four ounces, or two to four primary protein units.

I think it is useful in therapy to instruct patients in a meal-planning system early in the course of therapy and then have them complete meal plans on a daily basis. These should be reviewed at regular intervals in therapy. In particular, if patients deviate from the plan, they should make changes in a different color ink on the plan so that both you and they can follow the areas in which they are having the most difficulty and the most success. Certain patients will have a lot of difficulty with certain food units. For example, one may find that she consistently overeats in the vegetable section, but has difficulty getting an adequate number of satiety units. If this problem is highlighted by the therapist, it will be easier for the patient to identify possible sources of satiety units and to make the necessary amendments in her pattern.

We now turn to dietary guidelines to teach patients as part of therapy. The guidelines provide a total daily Kcal intake of 1,450 to 1,700 Kcal, depending on whether the lowest or highest number of units are selected. This level of Kcal provides an intake range that is adequate for about 90% of our patients. Shorter and/or less active patients can be instructed in the smaller amounts, taller and/or more active in the larger amounts. With those who are highly atypical (very tall, competitive athlete), it is best to get input from a dietician. Most importantly, the patient needs to be taught that the only way to really find out what she needs to eat is trial and error, unless you have access to an apparatus to repeatedly measure resting energy expenditure, a very useful technique, but one that is expensive, logistically difficult to arrange, and not widely available.

If the patient consistently gains weight, you can discuss how best to cut back, and if she loses weight, how to increase intake.

VII. General Guidelines

A. Eat three meals each day. Do not skip meals for any reason. If you binge and purge during the day, eat a meal as usual at the next scheduled time.

B. Designate regular meal times and eat your meals within one hour of those designated times. Avoid going more than six hours between breakfast and lunch and lunch and dinner. If long periods of time are unavoidable between meals, plan a snack to avoid becoming overly hungry.

C. Plan your meals in advance to reduce the anxiety of making food choices and assure that the foods you need will be available.

D. Keep records of your actual intake and compare it regularly with the recommendations provided.

E. Weigh yourself no more than once a week. Do this at the same time of day in the same type of clothing.

F. Include some meat, fish, poultry, or milk at each meal.

G. Limit raw vegetables (especially lettuce) and sugar-free gum to prevent early satiety and bloating.

H. Be sure to get six to eight cups of caffeine-free beverages such as water, milk, juice, soup, etc., daily. Although caffeine-containing beverages such as coffee, tea, and colas are also permitted, limit these to one serving per meal to assure that you eat all the health foods recommended.

I. Intake should include:

4–5 units primary protein: Lean meat, fish, or poultry. Generally 1 unit=1 ounce.

This includes meat, fish, and skinless poultry prepared by roasting, broiling, or boiling. If foods are fried, subtract 1 unit satiety (1 tsp. butter/margarine) for each one eaten. Additional substitutions for one unit include 1 egg, 1 once low-fat cheese, 1/4 cup tuna or 1/4 cup low-fat cottage cheese. Two tbsp. of peanut butter count as 1 unit of primary protein and 2 satiety units (2 tsp. butter/margarine).

5–6 units satiety factor: Butter, margarine or oil. 1 unit=1 tsp.

Additional substitutions include 1 tbsp. cream cheese; 1 tbsp. French, Italian, or thousand island salad dressing; 1/2 tbsp. mayonnaise; or 2 tbsp. coffee cream.

6–7 units of cereal and energy-rich vegetables: 1 unit=1 slice bread, 3/4 cup of ready-to-eat cereal, 1/2 cup of cooked cereal, 1/2 cup rice or pasta.

Energy-rich vegetables include corn, peas, cooked dried beans, potatoes, winter squash, sweet potatoes, or yams. one unit of energy-rich vegetables equals about 1/2 cup.

1–2 units of vegetables: 1 unit=1 cup.

This includes all except the energy-rich vegetables. If vegetables are prepared with butter/margarine, omit 1 tsp. satiety unit for each 1/2 cup of vegetables.

5–6 units of fruit or fruit juice: 1 unit=1 small apple; 1/2 banana; 1 average peach, pear, or orange; 1/2 cup mixed fruit or fruit juice.

2–4 units of calcium-rich foods: I recommend skim milk. 1 unit=1 cup.

Substitutions for skim milk include Alba 77® breakfast drink or cocoa and nonfat unflavored yogurt. Omit one unit satiety for each unit of 2% milk. Most fruit-flavored low-fat yogurts are equivalent to 1 unit skim milk, 1 unit satiety, and 1 unit fruit per 8-ounce portion.

For Day:			Name:						
			FOOD VALUE						
	FOOD ITEM	AMOUNT	PRIMARY PROTEIN	SATIETY FOODS	GRAIN/ ENERGY VEGIES	VEGIES	FRUITS	CALCIUM- RICH FOODS	FLUIDS
TIME									
B R E A K F A S T									
TIME									
L U N C H									
TIME									
D I N N E R									
TOTAL NUMBER OF FOOD UNITS (LISTED ABOVE)									
INDIVIDUALIZED MEAL PATTERN ("Goal for the Day")									

Figure 4. Meal Plan Form

A form for planning meals based on this system is shown as figure 4. A more comprehensive listing of food equivalents, called the Healthy Eating Food Lists, can be ordered from the Eating Disorders Program, University of Minnesota, Department of Psychiatry, Box 301, 420 Delaware Street S.E., Minneapolis, MN 55455.

VIII. Some patients find it easier at first to follow a specific meal plan supplied to them. However, the long-term goal is for the patient to learn to plan her own meals. What follows are sample meal plans, again designed to provide weight maintenance for a young woman of average height. I have used standard units of measurement rather than food units here, since this may be easier for some patients initially.

Day One	Day Two
1 cup grapefruit juice	1/2 large cantaloupe
1 bagel	4 rice cakes
2 tbsp. cream cheese	2 tbsp. peanut butter
1 Alba drink	1 Alba drink
Coffee, tea, or water	Coffee, tea, or water
1/2 cup cottage cheese	Tuna salad sandwich:
1 cup pineapple	1 cup tuna
6 rye crisp crackers	1 tbsp. mayonnaise
1 cup carrot and celery sticks	2 slices wheat bread
Coffee, tea, or water	1 large apple
	Coffee, tea, or water
2–3 oz. turkey	1 broiled chicken breast
1/2 cup rice	1 medium potato
1/2 cup broccoli	1/2 cup carrots
1 small roll	2 tsp. butter or margarine
1 medium apple	1 banana
1 cup skim milk	Coffee, tea, or water
Coffee, tea or water	

Day Three

1 1/2 cups Special K®
1 medium banana
1 cup skim milk
Coffee, tea, or water

Salad:
    1/2 cup lettuce
    1/2 cup raw vegetables
    2 tbsp. sunflower seeds
    2 tbsp. French dressing
    2 oz. grated cheese
1 medium, soft bread stick
1 cup cider
Coffee, tea, or water

2-3 oz. broiled haddock
1/2 cup potatoes
1/2 cup mixed vegetables
1 dinner roll
2 tsp. butter or margarine
1 cup fresh grapes
1 cup skim milk
Coffee, tea, or water

Day Four

8 oz. fruited low-fat yogurt
1 medium bran muffin
Coffee, tea, or water

Turkey sandwich:
    2 oz. turkey
    1/2 tbsp. mayonnaise
    2 slices wheat bread
    lettuce and tomato
1 medium orange
Coffee, tea, or water

Stir-fry chicken and vegetables:
    1/2 boneless chicken breast
    1 cup Chinese vegetables
    1 tbsp. oil
1 cup rice
1 medium apple
1 cup skim milk
    Coffee, tea, or water

Day Five

1 cup orange juice
2 slices wheat toast
2 tbsp. peanut butter
1 cup skim milk
Coffee, tea, or water

Day Six

2 grapefruit halves
1 cup granola cereal
1 cup skim milk
Coffee, tea, or water

Chef salad:
  1 oz. cheese
  1 oz. ham
  1/2 cup lettuce
  1 cup raw vegetables
  2 tbsp. French dressing
1 medium, soft bread stick
1 cup fresh fruit
Coffee, tea, or water

Stuffed baked potato:
  1–2 oz. grated cheese
  1 medium baked potato
  1/2 cup broccoli
1 cup fruited low-fat yogurt
Coffee, tea, or water

2 english muffin halves
2 oz. melted cheese
1 medium apple
Coffee, tea, or water

Frozen Dinner— < 300 Kcal
(Lean Cusine,® etc.)
1 small dinner roll
1 tsp. butter or margarine
1 medium banana
1 cup skim milk
Coffee, tea, or water

Day Seven

1 cup grapefruit juice
1 medium bran muffin
1 cup skim milk
Coffee, tea, or water

Tuna salad sandwich:
  1/2 cup tuna
  1 tbsp. mayonnaise
  2 slices wheat bread
  lettuce and tomato
1 cup fresh grapes
Coffee, tea, or water

Broiled chicken breast
1 cup white and wild rice
1 cup carrots
2 tsp. butter or margarine
1 medium apple
1 cup skim milk
Coffee, tea, or water

Day Eight

1 cup oatmeal
1/4 cup raisins
1 cup skim milk
Coffee, tea, or water

2 soft tacos:
  2 small flour tortillas
  1 oz. lean ground beef
  1/4 cup grated cheese
  lettuce and tomato
  taco sauce
1 medium orange
Coffee, tea, or water

2-3 oz. broiled salmon
1 medium baked potato
2 tsp. butter or margarine
1/2 cup broccoli
1 cup fresh fruit
1 Alba® drink
Coffee, tea, or water

Day Nine	Day Ten

Day Nine

1 cup fruited low-fat yogurt
1 medium bran muffin
Coffee, tea, or water

Ham sandwich:
  1 oz. lean ham
  1/2 tsp. mayonnaise
  2 slices whole-grain bread
  lettuce and tomato
1 package Fruit Wrinkles®
Coffee, tea, or water

Frozen dinner:
  (Lean Cuisine,® Dining Lite,®
  etc. < 300 Kcals)
1 crescent roll and 1 tsp. butter
  or margarine
1 cup sparkling cider
1 cup skim milk
Coffee, tea, or water

Day Ten

1 cup orange juice
1 1/2 cup Special K®
1 cup skim milk
Coffee, tea, or water

1 small hamburger
1 small serving french fries
1 medium apple
Coffee, tea, or diet drink

Pasta salad:
  1 cup pasta
  1/2 cup chicken or tuna
  1 cup raw vegetables
  1 tbsp. mayonnaise
8 oz. fruited low-fat yogurt
Coffee, tea, or water

8

Pharmacotherapy of Bulmia Nervosa

One of the true success stories in clinical neurosciences over the last 30 or so years has been the development of effective drug therapies of several psychiatric disorders. This era was heralded by the introduction of chlorpromazine for the treatment of schizophrenia in the early 1950s. Since that time, drug therapy has come to play an important part in the treatment of many emotional and behavioral disorders, several of which were previously difficult or impossible to treat. These include schizophrenia, affective disorders, obsessive compulsive disorder, and other anxiety disorders. Therefore, it is logical and important to attempt to find medications that will be effective in bulimia nervosa, and several research groups have focused their attention in this area.

There are two other specific reasons why drug treatments for bulimia nervosa have been pursued. First, many patients with bulimia nervosa demonstrate symptoms suggestive of other psychiatric disorders, particularly affective disorders.[183] This overlap or comorbidity has led some researchers to conceptualize eating disorders as variants of affective disorders.[184] (See chapter 3 for a summary of this line of reasoning.) Valid or not, the hypothesis is a useful one in that it has generated much discussion and meaningful research. Second, as was summarized in the discussion of psychobiology, researchers increasingly have begun to unravel the basic biological mechanisms, both central and peripheral, that control eating and appetite, and some of this research has suggested pharmacological strategies that can be used to modify eating behavior in humans.[322]

The pharmacological research on bulimia nervosa to date has been quite promising, and suggests that many patients with bulimia nervosa will benefit from such interventions; however, as we will see, many problems remain, the most important being the identification of those patients for whom pharmacotherapy is desirable, as opposed to those patients for whom psychotherapy, or perhaps no therapy at all, may be preferable. We will return to this and other related questions after discussing some of the specific agents that have been used experimentally.

Antidepressant Treatments of Bulimia Nervosa

Pope, Hudson, and their colleagues at MacClean Hospital were the first to suggest and then to demonstrate the utility of tricyclic antidepressants in the treatment of bulimia nervosa,[359,360] and Walsh and colleagues at Columbia University the first to suggest and demonstrate the utility of MAO (monoamine oxidase) inhibitors.[459,460] Since these reports, a series of nine placebo-controlled, double-blind trials, wherein controls were used to guard against investigator bias, have been reported in the medical literature.[6,14,29,176,196,299,362,391,456]

I will first discuss the methodology used in these studies. Why are placebo controls — treating some of the subjects with an inactive drug — important? Placebo control groups are important because simply seeing a physician regularly and self-monitoring eating behavior will benefit some patients. Without adequate controls, it is impossible to know which treatment components (the drug, the doctor, the setting) are really therapeutic. Some subjects, therefore, receive drugs and others placebos, but the rest of the treatment conditions are identical. Also, such studies are 'blind,' that is, neither physicians nor subjects know whether any given patient is taking drug or placebo (although side-effects at times give it away); assignments are made randomly to further guard against investigator bias.

The controlled studies are summarized in tables 17 and 18. The first study, reported by Pope and colleagues,[362] used the tricyclic antidepressant imipramine, and found this antidepressant to be superior to placebo treatment in reducing the frequency of target eating behaviors, such as binge-eating and vomiting, as well as improving mood, as assessed using the Hamilton Depression Scale. In the second study, mianserin,[391] an antidepressant not currently marketed in the United States, was used. Sabine and colleagues failed to demonstrate a significant advantage for the active drug. One possible explanation is that the dosage may have been subtherapeutic. Our group subsequently reported a placebo-controlled, double-blind trial of amitriptyline.[299] We also found significant improvement on

Table 17. Overview of Controlled Antidepressant Treatment Studies in Bulimia Nervosa

Year	Author	Drug	Dosage	Design	Duration	Reduction Binge-Eating[a]
1983	Pope et al.	Imipramine	200 mg	Parallel	6 wk.	70%
1983	Sabine et al.	Mianserin	60 mg	Parallel	8 wk.	
1984	Mitchell & Groat	Amitriptyline	150 mg	Parallel	8 wk.	72%
1986	Hughes et al.	Desipramine	200 mg	Parallel	6 wk.	91%
1987	Agras et al.	Imipramine	$\bar{x}=167$ mg	Parallel	16 wk.	72%
1988	Walsh et al.	Phenelzine	69–90 mg	Parallel	8 wk.	64%
1988	Barlow et al.	Desipramine	150 mg	Crossover	6 wk.	
1988	Horne et al.	Bupropion	450 mg	Parallel	8 wk.	67%
1988	Blouin et al.	Desipramine	150 mg	Crossover	6 wk.	
		Fenfluramine	60 mg			

[a]Mean reduction in frequency of binge-eating for patients on active drug.

placebo, but numerically more improvement on active drug, although on most eating variables there was only a statistical trend favoring the active treatment. However, on mood variables there was a clear significant advantage for active drug over placebo.

Hughes and colleagues[196] at the Mayo Clinic subsequently reported a placebo-controlled, double-blind trial using desipramine, again demonstrating an advantage for active drug over placebo on both mood and eating variables. This study was unique in two respects. First, patients who did not meet criteria for major depressive disorder were used in an attempt to examine whether or not the effectiveness of the drug was dependent on a concomitant depression problem. The authors found that the drug worked quite well, despite the absence of depression. Second, serum levels were carefully monitored, and patients who initially were nonresponders had their levels titrated into a therapeutic range. Many of these patients subsequently responded. Walsh and colleagues[456] reported a significant advantage for the MAO inhibitor phenelzine compared to the placebo in a double-blind, placebo-controlled trial, and Agras and associates[6] reported a significant advantage for imipramine over the placebo in another study. Most recently, three additional trials, two using desipramine,[14,28] and one using bupropion,[176] have appeared, all indicat-

Table 18. Involvement, Completion, and Outcomes in Controlled Antidepressant Treatment Studies

Author(s)	Drug	Drug or Placebo	Started	Did Not Complete	Completed	% Reduction BE Frequency Pre-to-Post-Rx[a]	% Abstinent last week of Rx
Pope et al.	Imipramine	D	11	2 (18%)	9 (82%)	70%	0%
		P	11	1 (9%)	10 (91%)	0%	0%
Sabine et al.	Mianserin	D	20	6 (30%)	14 (70%)		
		P	30	8 (27%)	22 (73%)		
Mitchell & Groat	Amitriptyline	D	21	5 (24%)	16 (76%)	72%	19%
		P	17	1 (6%)	16 (94%)	52%	19%
Hughes et al.	Desipramine	D	10	3 (30%)	7 (79%)	91%	68%
		P	12	3 (25%)	9 (75%)	19%	
Agras et al.	Imipramine	D	10	0 (0%)	10 (100%)	72%	30%
		P	12	2 (17%)	10 (83%)	43%	10%
Walsh et al.	Phenelzine	D	31	8 (26%)	23 (74%)	64%	35%
		P	31	4 (13%)	27 (88%)	5%	4%
Barlow et al.	Desipramine	D	47	23 (49%)	24 (51%)	4%	
Horne et al.	Bupropion	D	55	18 (33%)	37 (68%)	67%	30%
		P	26	14 (54%)	12 (46%)	2%	0%
Blouin et al.	Desipramine Fenfluramine	D	36	14 (39%)	22 (61%)		

[a]Mean reduction in frequency of binge-eating for patients on active drug.

ing benefit for the antidepressant. Taken together, these studies document effectiveness for antidepressants compared to placebos.

There are several other considerations that are important. First, there was a marked difference in placebo response rate across these studies, varying from no placebo response to 52% reduction in the frequency of target behaviors. This suggests differences between samples or difference in the supportive psychotherapy, an inherent component in medication management, that is delivered along with the medication. Second, most of these studies have been of short duration, and there are questions about the durability of improvement. To my knowledge, there has only been one long-term follow-up drug study published, a report by Pope and colleagues of a two-year follow-up of the original sample of patients treated in their imipramine trial.[361] They found that although some patients could be effectively withdrawn from medication and maintain their improvement, a sizable subgroup relapsed without medication, and many required several medication changes or adjustments to maintain remission. In short, the management of these patients over time was not an easy task, even for skilled physicians knowledgeable in the drug treatment of bulimia nervosa. Third, in all of the drug studies reported, there has been a significant and usually dramatic decrement in the frequency of target behaviors. However, the percentage of patients who were free of symptoms at the end of treatment is surprisingly low in most studies. Therefore patients are improved but many are not "cured." Fourth, the mechanism of the drug effect is unclear. There does not appear to be a clear relationship between the presence of depression and drug effectiveness, as illustrated by Hughes and colleagues,[196] Horne and colleagues,[176] and our study,[299] which stratified for depression. Depression actually seems to be a negative predictor for drug response, in that patients who are most depressed tend to do least well.

The relative efficacy of MAO inhibitors and tricyclic antidepressants in this condition remains to be determined, and both classes have potential advantages and disadvantages because of their side effects, which we will review later.

Lithium Carbonate

Hsu in 1984 reported an open-label (nonblind) trial using lithium in 14 outpatients with bulimia nervosa.[178] Of these patients, 8 were also receiving cognitive-behavioral therapy, and 6 had been failures in cognitive-behavioral therapy. The improvement rates were quite impressive on the drug, with 12 of the 14 patients showing at least a 75% reduction in binge-eating behavior. Hsu recently reported another six-week open-label trial using lithium in 17 additional patients, again in combination with cognitive-behavioral therapy. Eleven showed at least a 75% reduction in symptom frequency, while 6 demonstrated less than a 50% reduction in target symptoms. Hsu concluded that, in the absence of double-blind trials, the utility of lithium is open to question, but that his experience suggests that lithium may be of benefit to some of these patients. However, lithium should be used cautiously in eating disorder patients, given the fluid and electrolyte abnormalities to which they are prone.

Anticonvulsants

We have previously discussed the work of Green, Rau and their colleagues concerning the possibility of EEG abnormalities underlying compulsive eating disorders.[137,374,375,376] These same authors treated a series of patients with the anticonvulsant phenytoin and in their initial report of the results noted that 9 of 10 patients responded quite well to the drug.[137] In a review of their work in this area, these authors reported that overall, 70% of 30 patients with abnormal EEGs improved on phenytoin, while only 35% of 17 patients with normal EEGs responded, suggesting efficacy for the drug in the subgroup of patients with the EEG abnormalities.

Wermuth and colleagues conducted a 12-week, double-blind crossover study, the results of which unfortunately were confounded.[470] In the phenytoin-placebo sequence, 5 of 10 patients were at least moderately improved on active drug, while in the placebo-phenytoin sequence 4 showed at least moderate improvement. However, there was a persistence of the positive treatment effect in the placebo period after the initial phenytoin treatment, and abnormal EEGs were documented in only 3 subjects.

The anticonvulsant carbamazepine, which has been shown recently to be effective in treating certain affective disorders, has also been used in some patients with bulimia nervosa. Kaplan and colleagues[230] reported they had treated a total of 16 patients with this drug in a double-blind, crossover study that was, at the time of their report, still in progress. The project included six-week periods, the sequences being carbamazepine/placebo/carbamazepine or placebo/carbamazepine/placebo for the first 6 patients, with only two of the six-week intervals being used for the last 10 patients. There was no difference overall in response to the active drug compared to placebo, although one patient appeared to have a complete remission and another a clear decrease in binge-eating and vomiting, with 3 others showing lesser degrees of improvement. These authors concluded that there may be a subgroup of bulimic patients who respond to this drug, and indicated that they would attempt to delineate such a subgroup in more detail in future research.

In summary, at this point one must conclude that evidence concerning the effectiveness of anticonvulsants in bulimia nervosa is mixed; and that the database on which to draw firm conclusions is inadequate; but that there is no convincing evidence for a correlation between seizure disorders, EEG abnormalities, and bulimia nervosa, or for efficacy in most of these patients, although interest in this area remains.

Opiate Antagonists in Bulimia

There is considerable interest in the role of brain chemical neurotransmitter systems in the control of eating. One such system, the endogenous opioid (opiatelike) peptide system, appears to be quite important in the control of feeding behavior in both human and infrahuman species, and there is evidence linking certain types of feeding, in particular stress-induced feeding, to this system.[307,321,324] Based on these observations, a few groups of investigators have attempted to use opiate antagonists to suppress binge-eating behavior in patients with bulimia.

Jonas and Gold first reported that the long-acting, orally active narcotic antagonist naltrexone hydrochloride was effective in reducing binge-eating and vomiting behavior in an open-label (nonblind) trial in 5 outpatients with bulimia nervosa.[220] Our group subsequently reported that the administration of naloxone, the short-acting opiate antagonist that requires parenteral administration, attenuated the amount of food eaten during binge-eating episodes in bulimic subjects hospitalized on a metabolic research ward.[306]

Jonas and Gold have continued to expand their series and have recently summarized their results in the treatment of 25 patients.[221] All had a prior incomplete response or lack of response to a trial of a tricyclic antidepressant. Five could not tolerate the naltrexone, but the other 20 subjects showed a dramatic and significant response when treated with 200 to 300 mg per day. One subject evidenced liver function abnormalities that cleared after a dosage reduction.

Our group has recently completed a placebo-controlled, double-blind trial of the long-acting orally active drug naltrexone in outpatients with bulimia nervosa (unpublished data). The study used a crossover design with a 50 mg dosage of naltrexone at bedtime. Subjects were initially put through a single-blind placebo phase to eliminate early placebo responders. Those who failed to improve significantly during the initial phase were then randomized to either the active drug or placebo and, following three weeks of therapy, crossed over to the other treatment. The results failed to demonstrate a statistical superiority for naltrexone compared to placebo on any of the important variables examined, although numerically the outcome favored naltrexone. A crossover study using 120 mg per day in 10 subjects found similar results.[201]

How do we reconcile the results of these last two studies with the work of Jonas and Gold? There are several important points here: First is the issue of dosage. Jonas and Gold have been employing dosages two to six times those used in the two controlled studies. We had initially selected the lower dose strategy because of the possibility of hepatotoxicity with this drug at high dosages. However, the prior research, which showed a risk for developing liver function abnormalities when subjects were treated with naltrexone, involved individuals who had obesity or Alzheimer's disease, not bulimia nervosa, and it remains to be seen whether or not naltrexone at high dosage can be used chronically and safely with bulimia patients. Jonas and Gold reported few problems in this regard. Second is the issue of the effect of the drug. While 50 mg a day of naltrexone is effective in blocking the effects of exogenously administered opiates, it may be insufficient to block certain endogenous opioids. An alternative hypothesis is that at high doses the drug exerts important effects in the control of eating that are not directly mediated through the endogenous opioid system. This remains to be examined further, perhaps in animal models.

Overall, at this point it seems most reasonable to conclude that there is some evidence that naltrexone at high dosages is useful in the treatment of some patients with bulimia nervosa. However, further work needs to be done in documenting which patients will respond and whether or not there is a risk, perhaps an excessive risk, of developing hepatotoxicity. It is particularly interesting that most of the patients used in the studies by Jonas and Gold had been tricyclic nonresponders, suggesting that they may constitute a special subgroup who responds to opioid blockade.

Other Drug Therapies

As reviewed in the chapter on psychobiology, serotonergic mechanisms appear to facilitate satiety responses in the periventricular and ventral medial hypothalamus. Therefore it seems reasonable to speculate that augmentation of serotonin may induce satiety and suppress eating in bulimic subjects. Krahn and I[250] reported in 1984 that we had attempted to use tryptophan to suppress eating behavior in these patients. One gram of tryptophan administered orally three times a day failed to have a significant effect on binge-eating behavior in a series of 13 patients with bulimia nervosa in a double-blind study. However, the small sample size and the fact that only one dosage was employed limit the interpretability of this study. The dose may have been subtherapeutic.

Fenfluramine is a drug that also facilitates serotonin transmission. Robinson and colleagues[380] reported the results of a single-dose administration study of fenfluramine 60 mg or placebo on eating behavior in a series of 15 bulimic patients. Fenfluramine significantly reduced food intake compared to placebo. None of the eating behavior demonstrated by the patients postfenfluramine was rated as a binge, while 6 of the 15 postplacebo administration meals were rated as nearly or definitely binges. Ong and colleagues demonstrated similar results using methylamphetamine infusions.[341]

The nontricyclic antidepressant fluoxetine is also being evaluated experimentally in the treatment of bulimia nervosa, and the results to date have been very promising. The drug is a very potent, specific serotonin re-uptake inhibitor and on theoretical grounds may be particularly helpful for these patients. An open-label, uncontrolled trial reported by Freeman and colleagues in 1985[114] found dramatic effects for the drug. Because the drug is not sedative for most patients and free of anticholinergic properties, it is a particularly desirable agent to consider in patients with bulimia nervosa.

Clinical Use of Drug Therapy for Bulimia Nervosa

When a physician is considering using drug therapy for this disorder, several questions need to be considered, and several things need to be asked of the patient.

First, is drug therapy an acceptable form of therapy *for* this patient? Put another way, is there any reason — medical or otherwise — why drugs may not be a safe approach? Certain drugs, such as the more highly anticholinergic tricyclics, should be avoided in patients with certain types of heart disease, for example. Fortunately, the medical conditions that preclude the safe use of these drugs are rare among bulimic patients, and the safety record of antidepressants in the population is impressive. Second, given proper education, is drug therapy an acceptable form of treatment *to* this patient? Some patients find the notion of drug treatment aversive, and if this bias cannot be dispelled by the physician or therapist, then these patients are unlikely to have the prescription filled, let alone take the drug on a regular basis. Therefore the second step must be is to assess the patient's motivation to take the medication.

Which patients will respond to drug treatment? Unfortunately, very few data are available about this. Response does not appear to be linked to depression—indeed nondepressed patients appear to do quite well on antidepressant drugs in terms of their eating behavior. Unfortunately, no specific variables have been delineated that are linked to response to antidepressant treatment in this population. Therefore, whether or not to use drug therapy is a matter of clinical judgment. Obviously this is a matter of considerable debate, and strong arguments can be made on both sides. Those who advocate the use of antidepressants can make the case that medications can be administered easily and are widely available, and that a sizable subgroup of patients respond dramatically to them. Also, such drugs are relatively inexpensive and take much less time for both therapist and patient than most forms of psychotherapy. However, those opposed to drug therapy can point out that antidepressants are unacceptable to some patients, that the side effects can be problematic, and that, particularly in patients who are significantly depressed, there is the risk of overdose. Psychotherapy advocates can also point out that many patients treated with antidepressants are improved but not free of the symptoms at the end of treatment. However, this criticism also can be leveled at many of the psychotherapy studies.

My current practice is to prescribe antidepressants as part of the initial treatment for patients who give a clear history of an affective disorder, in particular if there is evidence that the affective disorder preceded the onset of the eating disorder, for patients who remain depressed despite improvement in their eating symptoms, and for those patients who show only a partial response or a lack of response to a psychotherapy intervention, whether or not they are depressed. I currently favor using a structured psychotherapy approach as the initial intervention for the rest, in hopes

Table 19. Overview of Available Heterocyclic Antidepressants

Drug	Therapeutic Dosage	t 1/2[a]	Sedation	Anti-cholinergic
Imipramine (Tofranil®)	150–300 mg	10–15	2+	2+
Desipramine (Norpramine®)	150–300 mg	20–25	1+	1+
Amitriptyline (Elavil®)	100–300 mg	20–30	3+	3+
Nortriptyline (Aventyl®)	75–100 mg	35–45	2+	1+
Protriptyline (Vivactil®)	40–60 mg	72–170	0-1+	3+
Doxepin (Sinequan®)	200–300 mg	18–30	4+	2+
Trimipramine (Surmontil®)	150–300 mg	8	3+	2+
Maprotiline (Ludiomil®)	150–300 mg	27–58	3+	(+)
Amoxapine (Ascendin®)	200–400 mg	30	3+	(+)
Trazodone (Desyrel®)	200–600 mg	13	2+	(+)
Fluoxetine (Prozac®)	20–60 mg	96	0	0

[a] + 1/2 = half-life

that such therapy will exert a prophylactic effect and prevent relapse or recurrences.

We will now turn to the practical aspects of antidepressant therapy. Many of the antidepressants that can be used in the treatment of bulimia nervosa are summarized in table 19 with some descriptive information. The MAO inhibitors will be discussed separately. Several of these antidepressant drugs have not yet been studied experimentally in bulimia nervosa. However, experience suggests that recently introduced drugs are beneficial despite the absence of large controlled trials.[185] Whether one or more will be found to be particularly effective remains to be seen.

Although loosely referred to as "tricyclics," the last five compounds on the list actually do not have the traditional three-ring molecular structure of most tricyclics. The last two, trazodone and fluoxetine, have very different chemical structures from the others, and because of this, different side-effect profiles. Also listed in table 19 are the usual therapeutic ranges for these drugs. It is important to keep these guidelines in mind, since a major cause for lack of response to antidepressants, whether one is treating depression or bulimia nervosa, is inadequate dosage. The third column reviews the relative sedative properties of the drugs. Some, such as amitriptyline and doxepin, are very sedative, while others, such as protriptyline and fluoxetine, lack sedative properties for most patients. In certain situations sedation may be desirable, particularly in a patient who is having marked sleep difficulties. At other times it is undesirable, particularly if it interferes with daytime functioning. The fourth column summarizes the relative anticholinergic effects of these drugs. Several of the drugs are very potent in antagonizing acetylcholine in the brain and periphery, such as imipramine and amitriptyline, while several of the newer compounds, particularly trazodone and fluoxetine, have few or no anticholinergic properties. This is important, in that anticholinergic effects are undesirable. They include dry mouth, constipation, blurred vision, and the possibility of conduction abnormalities and arrhythmias in individuals with preexisting organic heart disease.

The major side effects of the traditional tricyclic compounds are summarized in table 20 by organ system. We have already mentioned sedation. Tremor is unusual. Confusion is unusual in young women with bulimia nervosa, but a significant problem in the elderly if they are treated with the highly anticholinergic antidepressants; those agents should be avoided in treating the elderly. Cardiovascular effects can result in hypotension and the possibility of cardiac rhythm disturbances in those with preexisting heart problems. Of the traditional tricyclics, desipramine and nortriptyline appear to be particularly safe in terms of hypotension, but still cause significant hypotension in some individuals. The endocrinological abnormalities and the hematologic abnormalities are quite rare. Also these drugs can make some patients more anxious and agitated and, when used to treat manic-depressive patients during a depressive phase, can precipitate manic psychotic episodes.

There are other differences among these drugs that make some more or less desirable. Maprotiline, for example, is quite safe as to its anticholinergic effects, but has a particular propensity to lower seizure threshold. For this reason it is not one of my first choices. Amoxapine again has a favorable anticholinergic profile, but has an active metabolite that has neuroleptic, antipsychotic activity and for that reason this drug can cause neurological side effects. Therefore in my judgment, amoxapine is not a first-choice agent. Trazodone does not cause the tachycardia seen with many tricyclics, but can cause significant hypotension. Overall, fluoxetine is probably the best tolerated of these agents, with the major side effects being anxiety, nausea, sleeplessness, and rash.

Of the drugs on this list, I prefer using fluoxetine, desipramine, and nortriptyline because they are relatively low or lacking in both sedative and anticholinergic effects.

**Table 20. Side Effects/Adverse
Reactions—Tricyclics**

1. Neuro
   a. Sedation
   b. Confusion
   c. Tremors
2. C:V
   a. Hypotension
   b. Heart block
3. Endocrine
   a. Gynecomastia
   b. Galactorrhea
   c. Serum glucose changes
4. Anticholinergic
5. Psychiatric
   a. Anxiety
   b. Precipitate Psychosis
6. Heme
   a. Eosinophilia
   b. Agranulocytosis

The MAO inhibitors most commonly used in the United States are summarized in table 21. These agents are used less frequently because of the dietary restrictions required of patients taking them. However, Walsh and colleagues[456] have demonstrated that they can be used safely in this population if patients are educated about foods that they need to avoid and medications they cannot use while taking the drugs. Phenelzine is the agent that has been demonstrated experimentally to be effective in the treatment of bulimia nervosa[456] but tranylcypramine is also widely used. Many of the side effects that we discussed with the other antidepressants are also applicable to the MAO inhibitors, with a few differences. The MAO inhibitors tend to be low in their anticholinergic effects, which is an advantage, but they are quite potent in lowering blood pressure, which makes them intolerable for some patients. Patients need to be very careful with their diet, since tyramine-containing food must be avoided, a difficult task for some bulimic patients. We use both phenelzine and tranylcypramine in our clinic quite commonly with bulimic patients and have had good success with both.

The clinical use of these drugs in bulimia nervosa resembles the clinical use of antidepressants for other conditions. The patient should be educated

Table 21. Overview of Available Monoamine Oxidase Inhibitors

Drug	Dosage	Latency	MAO Substrate
Hydrazine			
Isocarboxazid (Marplan®)	10–30 mg	3–4 wks.	Type A & B
Phenelzine (Nardil®)	15 tid to 90 mg/day	3–4 wks.	Type A & B
Nonhydrazine			
Tranylcypramine (Parnate®)	20–60 mg	10 days	Type A & B

as to the possible side effects of the drug, in particular that with most agents they can expect some mild sedation and possibly constipation. They also should be educated about the delay of onset of action, which is often two to three weeks, so that they do not become discouraged and discontinue the drug. Also, the need to take the medication faithfully and carefully follow the dosage adjustments must be stressed, as some patients assume that they should take these drugs only when they feel upset or particularly depressed.

When I am prescribing nortriptyline, I usually start the patient on a dosage of 25 mg at bedtime, with instructions to increase to 50 mg three days later. I then see the patient in my office a few days later, check her vital signs, solicit data about side effects and toxicity and, if all is going as planned, increase her to 75 mg with instructions to increase to 100 mg three days later. I allow an adequate amount of time to approach steady state and then check the serum level of the drug. In using fluoxetine, I generally start with a dosage of 20 mg poqam and increase by one pill every two weeks until I see a response or reach 60 mg a day.

If patients do respond, the question then becomes, "How long should they be treated?" I previously discussed the work of Pope, Hudson and their colleagues. Their follow-up study, and my clinical experience, indicate that many patients need to take these drugs for long periods of time, at minimum six months to a year, and that some will require the drugs beyond that point if they are to remain in remission. Frankly, we need considerably more information about the course of bulimia nervosa and about maintenance therapies for this disorder before firm guidelines can be offered. Given the present state of knowledge, I think it is reasonable to try to taper antidepressant-responders off the drug after six to nine months of therapy, to see if the drug is still necessary.

9

General Treatment Considerations

There are many reasons to be optimistic about the treatment of patients with bulimia nervosa. Published treatment studies show quite clearly that most individuals with this disorder improve dramatically with therapy and that many apparently recover from the condition. However, there are important questions concerning treatment that we cannot yet answer, including the relative efficacy of various treatments and which treatments are best for which patients. We know even less about the possibility of long-term relapse following treatment, and the relative prophylactic effects of various interventions.

In this chapter we will review the published psychotherapy treatment studies of bulimia nervosa. But first, it is useful to consider several theoretical points, some posing dichotomous positions, that are conceptually important in the treatment of bulimia nervosa.

Self-Help Versus Formal Treatment

In recent years there has been a growth in the availability of self-help groups for individuals with bulimia nervosa. Although no reliable figures exist, it is reasonable to assume that a large number, perhaps the majority of individuals who seek help for this disorder, do so through involvement in self-help groups. The choice of a self-help approach probably rests on several considerations, including the unavailability of formal treatment service in many areas, problems in paying for treatment, and the desire to avoid the stigma of formal psychiatric care.

Several self-help approaches have been described in the literature.

Some were specifically designed for individuals with eating disorders, but many derived from techniques generated in other treatment or self-help contexts, such as Overeaters Anonymous (OA) or Alcoholics Anonymous (AA), and modified to address the particular needs of individuals with bulimia nervosa. Owing to the nature of self-help approaches, no outcome data have been published documenting the efficacy of such approaches or indicating the severity of the participants' symptoms. While one might assume that most bulimic individuals who participate in self-help organizations to improve their eating behavior are less ill than those seeking formal treatment, there is no information to substantiate this.

Although this book is directed toward professionals who encounter and at times treat bulimia nervosa, I will offer some general guidelines, based on experience rather than research, concerning involvement in self-help organizations.

1. Self-help groups in which most of the participants are actively bulimic usually are not helpful for bulimic individuals, and may actually perpetuate the problem. Such groups may provide a setting for support and encouragement, but may subtly encourage the symptoms of the disorder, if being symptomatic is the group norm. It is best to suggest to patients seeking self-help involvement that it be in the context of a group in which most of the members are in control of their eating behavior. In such a group they will have available the appropriate models for recovery.

2. Although some Overeaters Anonymous groups work well with people with bulimia nervosa, others do not. Also, there are certain philosophical issues in the OA view of eating problems that are at best unproductive and at worst countertherapeutic for many individuals with bulimia nervosa. (This will be discussed further when we talk about abstinence) Therefore, I think OA involvement needs to be considered on a group-by-group basis, and that therapists should not routinely refer patients to OA as a resource in the community.

Which individuals will do well with self-help groups, and which need formal treatment? Unfortunately we do not know; therefore, it is safest to recommend formal treatment when it is available.

Outpatient versus Inpatient Treatment

There has been a proliferation of inpatient treatment units for eating disorders in most metropolitan areas in the United States over the last decade. Some of this growth undoubtedly reflects a genuine concern for the welfare of these patients and a desire to implement innovative, effective treatment programs. But I believe that many of these facilities actually represent business decisions of hospital administrators who have been facing increasing problems with bed utilization. Regardless of the why these units have been developed, the central question is: Are they effective? As stressed by Vandereycken, this is an important research question.[448] However, all of the controlled treatment studies of bulimia nervosa of which I am aware have been conducted in outpatient settings, and it is clear that most patients with this disorder can be treated out of hospital. Certainly inpatient admission is desirable for certain individuals, but these situations are rare. Following are some possible reasons for hospital admission:

1. Lack of response to a formal, structured outpatient treatment specifically designed for bulimia nervosa. A period in the hospital may give such individuals an opportunity to gain control of their behavior, but such admissions should be brief.
2. The presence of a concomitant medical/psychiatric problem that precludes safe outpatient care. This would include medical instability and severe depression complicated by suicidal preoccupation.
3. The need for withdrawal from laxatives or diuretics. The complications of withdrawal, discussed in the section on medical complications and reviewed in the section on special treatment considerations, are so onerous for some patients that they will be unsuccessful unless they are in a closed environment where their access to the abused substances is restricted and they can be carefully observed.

There are also several reasons to avoid inpatient admissions whenever possible

1. The relative ease with which patients gain control of their eating behavior in a novel hospital environment. The frequent attention by staff and the absence of usual environmental cues make interruption of the behaviors quite likely. Unfortunately all too often these changes do not continue once the patient is back in the natural environment, faced with the usual stresses. In terms of learning theory, it is far superior for patients to gain control of their eating out of hospital, where they are dealing with the same internal and external cues that they will have to face after treatment.
2. Hospitalization is disruptive to patients and families, and there is

a certain personal and social stigma attached to having been hospitalized in a psychiatric setting.

3. Hospitalization is expensive and difficult to justify, given that cost-effective outpatient programs have been developed.

4. Working with inpatients may give members of a treatment staff a false sense of their own personal effectiveness, since patients often are compliant as inpatients, and appear to be highly motivated and doing well at discharge. Patients leave optimistic but often ill prepared for what they will face. Therefore, it is highly desirable for individuals who work with eating disorder patients in an inpatient setting to also be involved in their follow-up and aftercare, so as to better observe and appreciate the strengths and weaknesses of the system in which they work.

Structured versus Unstructured

Two central, related questions are the theoretical orientation of the therapist, and how the therapist views the symptoms of the disorder. Are the abnormal eating behaviors best viewed as symptomatic of an underlying psychological problem and, if so, should this underlying problem be the focus of therapy, while directing little attention to the behaviors per se;[473] or are the behaviors best viewed as significant components of the disorder that need to be addressed directly and early in the course of treatment?[101] Although many theoretical approaches have been suggested, usually favoring one or the other of these points of view, most approaches have not yet been tested experimentally.

A thorough review of all the published treatment observations and suggestions by practitioners of various theoretical schools is beyond the scope of this book, and interested readers are referred to the primary sources, several of which are included in the reference list. The bias of this text is toward behavioral and cognitive-behavioral approaches, with a strong emphasis on the interruption of the bulimic symptoms, supplemented by the use of psychopharmacological treatments with some patients.

Abrupt Abstinence versus Gradual Interruption of Target Behaviors

In the treatment literature for bulimia nervosa, an important, interesting debate has developed around this issue. The extremes of this debate are what we will call a *pure abstinence model* and a *pure cognitive-behavioral model*. The abstinence model has grown out of abstinence models applied to other types of problems, such as overeating (Overeaters Anonymous) and alcohol abuse (Alcoholics Anonymous). In such models the abnormal eating behavior is conceptualized as food abuse, from which the individual needs to be abstinent, and generally abstinence is required early in the course of treatment. Evidently many programs around the country have adopted this type of model, although we know little about their results since no systematic outcome studies have been published. The other extreme, the cognitive-behavioral therapy (CBT) approach, does not require abstinence from the behaviors and actually regards the presence of symptoms as desirable early in treatment to provide the individual an opportunity to learn from the episodes. The emphasis is more on understanding the behavioral and cognitive factors involved in the maintenance of the problems rather than their cessation. This dichotomy has been well described by Bemis.[17]

While our group at the University of Minnesota was an early advocate of an abstinence approach, we have increasingly moved in the direction of the cognitive-behavioral model which does not require abstinence, and have increasingly conceptualized problem eating behaviors as a positive opportunity to learn. In our current research efforts we are using what we call a *rapid interruption model*, which has some similarities to an abstinence model but also many elements used in most pure CBT approaches. We are now comparing this rapid interruption model to a pure CBT approach in research.

There are pros and cons for both a pure abstinence and a pure CBT model, as summarized by Bemis.[17] The main advantages of the abstinence model is that it gives patients clear-cut priorities, and it can be a very powerful motivating agent. The main problem is that it can teach patients a view of their symptoms that is not really valid, i.e., that "abstinence" is possible as an absolute, when we know from follow-up studies that many patients who have a very successful outcome long-term will have lapses of bulimic behavior and will at times overeat. Therefore "abstinence" is relative. Also, programs emphasizing abstinence may instill in patients a strong sense of guilt and shame, best exemplified by the practice of removing patients from group or individual therapy if they are unable to gain control of their eating behavior. This was once the practice in our clinic, and we eventually concluded that this was negative not only for pa-

Table 22. Comparison of Three Theoretical Approaches to Treatment of Bulimia Nervosa

Variable	Abstinence Model	Rapid Interruption Model	Pure CBT Model
Role of therapist	Variable or no therapist	Expert in eating disorders facilitator, often directive.	Expert in eating disorders, facilitator, but strong emphasis on teaching patients to "test" beliefs, assumption.
Role of insight	Not necessary to stop symptoms.	Desirable, but not necessary to stop symptoms.	Necessary for successful outcome
Meal planning	"Forbidden" foods and overeating to be avoided at all costs—will lead to relapse.	Meal planning based on appropriate intake strongly encouraged.	Meal planning based on appropriate intake strongly encouraged.
Feared/"forbidden" foods	Patients taught not to eat certain things, or more than a certain amount, because this will lead to a relapse.	Taught to incorporate and encouraged to reintroduce feared and forbidden foods; no foods excluded, but ok to avoid binge foods early.	Taught to incorporate and encouraged to reintroduce feared or forbidden foods; no foods excluded.
Attention to cognitions regarding food, weight	?	CBT techniques emphasized; however, patients encouraged to interrupt bulimic behaviors early in treatment.	Central focus of treatment.
Response of therapist to bulimic symptoms during treatment	Strongly negative—may lead to termination from therapy.	Seen as inevitable for some patients but not necessary or desirable for learning and, if frequent, discouraged and labeled as hazardous to adequate recovery.	Viewed as opportunity to learn; seen as a valuable part of treatment.
"Slips"	Seen as evidence of failure and, in some treatment programs, the equivalent of relapse.	Seen as quite common during the process of recovery and as an opportunity to learn, but accorded a negative valence.	Seen as likely and as an opportunity to learn; gives patients the opportunity to gather data during treatment.
Expectations of abstinence by end of treatment	Required.	Thought highly desirable—lack of abstinence seen as probably predictor of relapse.	Desirable but not necessary for success; continued improvement viewed as likely.

tients who left the group, but also for those who stayed. However, a pure CBT model presents other limitations and problems. The model can seem too theoretical and intellectual to some patients, and in general it is more difficult to motivate patients using this model, particularly early in treatment.

In table 22, I have summarized some of the basic ingredients in a pure abstinence program, in an intermediate program that I have called the *rapid interruption model,* and in a pure CBT model. No programs will exactly fit any of these three models, but many structured programs are similar to one of them. It is my opinion that the pure abstinence model is no longer tenable, given what we know about the longitudinal course of bulimia nervosa—that most patients will have symptoms during recovery and need to learn to understand and control them—and given the shame and guilt that can be associated with that approach. It seems to me that the more important question now is the relative efficacy of the other two types of programs. Can some elements of the abstinence model, in particular the use of a strong expectation for rapid interruption of symptoms early in treatment, serve as a powerful motivating variable for patients, yet not unduly encourage guilt and shame in those who are unsuccessful? These are important theoretical considerations and we need to gather more data before drawing any final conclusions.

Weight Extremes

A subgroup of patients with bulimia nervosa also meet criteria for anorexia nervosa, and a subgroup are quite overweight. We will discuss the former group first.

In most reported series of patients with anorexia nervosa, 45 to 50% of patients have bulimic symptoms.[26,55,90,423,424,425] This bulimic anorectic subgroup is particularly difficult to treat, in that they need to gain weight but also need to control their bulimic symptoms. Perhaps more common are bulimic patients who do not have sufficient weight loss to meet criteria for anorexia nervosa but who have many anorectic features (severe body-image distortion, constant preoccupation with weight loss, much fasting behavior).

These two subgroups are difficult to treat for several reasons. They are often younger than the average normal-weight bulimic patients and less mature. Many times, perhaps owing to their low weight, they are less able to cooperate effectively in treatment. Many also have poor insight into their illness. For these reasons, much of the primary treatment must be directed toward the anorexia nervosa features. These subgroups are not dealt with extensively in this book. However, many of the treatment concepts outlined here can be useful with these patients, although additional elements are necessary.

The group of overweight bulimia nervosa patients is less well understood. Some of these are individuals who gain weight owing to the bulimia nervosa, while others are overweight individuals who developed a bulimic eating pattern in an attempt to lose weight. Hudson and colleagues have shown that members of this overweight subgroup are less likely to vomit than normal-weight bulimics, but do have the same family loading for affective disorder.[191]

Most overweight bulimics want weight loss desperately and are highly resistant to following a regular balanced meal plan with adequate caloric intake. What level of caloric intake should we recommend for this group of patients? Should they maintain their body weight while attempting to control their eating? Clearly this would be unacceptable to many of them. Should they be placed on a weight-loss diet? This can be problematic; in my experience it is difficult if not impossible for patients to gain control of binging and vomiting when they are engaging in severely restrictive dieting. My approach is to place such patients on a meal plan that would maintain them at their ideal body weight; intake at this level will allow their weight to gradually drift toward a normal range without severely restrictive dieting.

Males With Bulimia Nervosa

One in 10 to 1 in 20 patients with bulimia nervosa are male.[10,298,328, 383,390,444] In most reported series, they are remarkably similar to women with the disorder in terms of age of onset and the duration of the illness prior to seeking treatment, and most of the treatment techniques we have discussed are equally applicable with males. However, there are several special considerations in treating male patients. First, there is much more of a social stigma attached to having bulimia nervosa if one is a male — this is perceived by the general public as an illness for girls and women, not men. Therefore men may be unwilling to seek treatment and, if looking for help, reticent to be treated in any program that might expose them to public view. The shame associated with having this condition should be discussed in therapy with these patients.

There is some information that the rate of homosexuality among men with bulimia nervosa is higher than the rate of homosexuality in the general population, although most men with bulimia nervosa are not gay.[164] However, the problems of being homosexual and the high valence placed on slimness, youth, and attractiveness in the homosexual subculture are important issues to discuss with gay male patients. Anecdotal information also suggests an association between athletic competition and training and the development of bulimia nervosa among men (e.g., gymnasts, wrestlers).[298]

Purging Other Than Vomiting

As we have seen, vomiting behavior is the usual method that bulimia patients use to rid themselves of excess calories. However, laxative and diuretic abuse are not uncommon and are, in my experience, particularly difficult to treat. Strong emphasis should be placed on interrupting these behaviors early in the course of the treatment, following the techniques we have outlined. If individuals are not able to stop using these substances, hospitalization to interrupt the cycle may be necessary. Three to five days in the hospital may allow the individual to gain control if they have been unable to do so outside.

Bulimia Nervosa Patients with Depression

As discussed, depression is very common in patients with bulimia nervosa.[183] However, the depression only rarely is so severe that patients cannot work productively in an outpatient structured psychotherapy program or cooperate with outpatient medication management. For patients who are seriously depressed, I think it is reasonable to initiate medication early in the course of treatment, but I continue to favor using structured behavioral techniques as the initial intervention with nondepressed patients, and the available data suggest that the two therapies can be used in tandem.

Bulimia Nervosa and Personality Disorders

The association between bulimia nervosa and significant personality disorders, particularly borderline personality disorder, remains a matter of considerable debate, and the literature estimates of the comorbidity for the two disorders vary dramatically, as we have seen.[214,271,358] There are some bulimic patients with severe personality disorder symptoms who will have difficulty participating meaningfully in structured outpatient behavioral/cognitive-behavioral psychotherapy, but in my experience the number of such patients is quite small. Many patients who have maladaptive personality disorder symptoms can still work effectively in therapy, if expectations are made clear and firm limits are set by the therapist. Some such patients cannot, but most can. I have also been increasingly impressed that what appear initially to be very dysfunctional personality traits may look quite different following the successful treatment of eating problems. Individuals appear more mature and better integrated and seem to have healthier interpersonal styles. Therefore I think there are problems in labeling patients as having a serious personality disorder when they are first evaluated for active bulimia nervosa.

Bulimia Nervosa and Drug/Alcohol Abuse

As we have discussed, the prevalence of drug and alcohol abuse problems in patients with bulmia nervosa is higher than expected for women in this age group, although the reasons for this remain unclear.[46,300] In clinical terms this is a significant problem, and not uncommmonly one encounters patients with both disorders. Considering the similarities between these conditions, I think it would be ideal to treat both conditions concurrently. However, I know of few programs that are able to do this effectively. Some chemical dependency treatment programs try, but most seem to be using a strict 12-step AA approach, which I believe is a less than optimal approach for bulimia nervosa.

The usual pattern in alcohol/drug abuse programs is not to address the eating disorder, focusing on the alcohol and drug abuse. Most bulimia nervosa treatment programs refer these dual-diagnosis patients for alcohol and drug abuse treatment first.

We originally speculated that some bulimic patients with a history of alcohol or drug abuse problems might have an activation of their drug use when their eating came under control, and I caution people about alcohol and drug use during and after treatment. However, I have not encountered this very often. It is useful, however, to point out to patients that it is not a good idea for them to use alcohol or drugs as a way of coping with the stress that is generated by attempting to control eating behavior.

Group versus Individual

Both group and individual approaches have their advocates, but no one has yet reported an adequate study of group versus individual psychotherapy using any of the theoretical models we have presented. Fairburn has argued that individual approaches are superior, particularly those using cognitive-behavioral techniques, since attention to each individual's problems can be included, while in group therapy individual issues to some extent have to be subsumed to the tasks of the group, particularly in short-term structured group approaches. However, there are possible advantages for group approaches. Patients can learn interpersonal skills through exposure and modeling with other patients and through practice in the group. The sense of altruism and shared learning that develops within a group, and recognition of common problems among patients, are also potential advantages of the group approach. However, in reality the list of determining variables in deciding between a group and individual approach usually is headed not by such considerations, but instead by issues of cost, availability, and the biases and training of the therapist. I think group therapy is an acceptable alternative for those patients whose psychopathology does not demand immediate, individual attention. Patients with severe personality disorders, such as borderline personality, probably fall into the latter category. However, we still need to determine which patient will do best in which type of therapy and, in particular, to identify that individual who will not function adequately in a group given her lack of interpersonal skills and other problems.

Bulimia Nervosa as a Syndrome versus a Recurrent Illness

Another interesting theoretical debate concerns our conceptualization of bulimia nervosa in the course of the affected individual's life. Some researchers have suggested a model, similar to that commonly applied to affective disorders, which predicts that bulimia nervosa is likely to recur, and therefore is likely to require prophylactic or repeated treatment, as do many patients with recurrent depression.[166] A different, in some ways opposite, model is that of bulimia nervosa as a behavioral disorder that can be time limited. The implications of this model would be that if an individual with bulimia nervosa understands her disorder, gains control of her behavior, and makes other necessary changes in her life, she can expect to be free of the disorder indefinitely. We have reviewed the published long-term outcome studies in chapter 1, and the data, far from clear, could be interpreted to support either of these models.

My stance in this debate, pending data to the contrary, is to sit on the fence and assume that bulimia nervosa may be a recurrent relapsing condition for some patients, particularly for those with concomitant depression, and a time-limited illness with little chance of relapse for others. I conceptualize bulimia nervosa as a behavioral disorder that can develop in those with few other problems or as a part of other recurrent or chronic medical (e.g., diabetes mellitus) or psychiatric (e.g., recurrent depression, borderline personality) conditions. In the former group I would predict a time-limited course; in the latter, a higher risk of recurrence. I find that it is difficult, however, to separate such groups at evaluation or early in treatment, except in extreme cases. It is also my experience that many individuals who initially look like candidates for a poor outcome do quite well, and that significant depressive problems or immature personality traits appear to resolve with improvement in eating. Therefore, I think that it best to tell patients that, while they may have problems later, the likelihood of relapse is probably low if they successfully complete a treatment program specifically designed for bulimia nervosa that incorporates relapse-prevention techniques. In treatment I favor an optimistic approach and I believe the available data support such optimism.

Controlled Psychotherapy Treatment Studies of Bulimia Nervosa

Beginning with the report of a group psychotherapy approach by Boskind-Lodahl and White in 1978[32] and 1981,[471] numerous approaches have been suggested in the literature. However, only 12 program reports have included some measure of scientific control, allowing an adequate assessment of the effectiveness of the therapy.[66,106,113,245,252,264,268,314,344,475,478,485] These programs and their comparison or control are summarized in table 23. As can be seen, most of the programs described have used group techniques, while two have employed individual forms of psychotherapy and four are classified as mixed, two using a combined individual and group approach, one comparing two individual approaches to a group approach, and one a group drug comparison. The programs have varied as to their duration and intensity, with most using a fixed schedule. Some have employed waiting-list controls, some minimal intervention controls, and four have compared other active treatments or modifications of the reference treatment.

Table 23. Overview of the Controlled Treatment Studies

Author(s)	Year	Active Treatment	Comparison or Control	Duration
		Group Therapy		
Connors et al.	1984	Pyschoeducational group	Waiting list	10 wk.
Yates & Sambrailo	1984	Group CBT + behavioral	Group CBT	6 wk.
Kirkley et al.	1985	Group CBT	Group nondirective	16 wk.
Lee & Rush	1986	Group CBT	Waiting list	6 wk.
Wilson et al.	1986	Cognitive restructuring ERP	Cognitive restructuring	16 wk.
Leitenberg et al.	1988	CBT + ERP (ms) CBT + ERP (ss) CBT	Waiting list	14 wk.
		Individual Therapy		
Ordman & Kirschenbaum	1985	Group full	Group brief	Variable
Fairburn et al.	1986	CBT	Individual short-term focal	18 wk.
		Mixed Therapy		
Lacey	1983	Individual + group	Waiting list	10 wk.
Freeman et al.	1985	Individual CBT Individual Behavioral Group	Waiting list	15 wk.
Wolchik et al.	1986	Psychoeducational group + Individual	Waiting List	7 wk.
Mitchell et al.	1988	Group CBT + Imipramine Group CBT + placebo Imipramine[a]	Placebo	12 wk.

[a]multiple vs. single settings
CBT – cognitive-behavioral therapy
ERP – exposure/response prevention
ms–multiple settings – single setting

In table 24, the numbers of patients who started treatment, dropped out or were withdrawn, and completed treatment are summarized. Also shown are treatment outcome data based on reduction of binge-eating behavior from baseline to posttreatment, as well as the percentage of patients who were free of bulimic symptoms for the last week of treatment. It must be remembered that this is only one of several ways to assess outcome, and many studies have omitted assessment of important areas of functioning. Wilson has reviewed outcome assessment in a recent paper.[476]

Although it might be assumed that the percentage of those free of symptoms at the end of treatment would be very important in assessing outcome, Fairburn has argued that patients treated using a CBT model actually continued to improve after treatment and that the percentage still demonstrating symptoms at the end of treatment is not crucial; indeed, his follow-up data support this hypothesis, as we will see.

Overall the reductions in the target behaviors such as binge-eating and in other symptoms such as vomiting (not shown) are fairly impressive and of the same order of magnitude as the reductions in frequencies reported by patients in the antidepressant drug studies for bulimia nervosa. However, as in the drug studies, many patients are continuing to have symptoms at the end of treatment. What this portends is difficult to know, and the small sample sizes and limited amount of data on long-term outcome, summarized in table 25, make it difficult to draw any firm conclusions. However, the available follow-up data do suggest that many patients are improved when followed up after treatment, and taken as a whole these studies suggest that programs specifically designed for the treatment of eating disorders have a higher degree of effectiveness than waiting lists or minimal interventions, illustrated by the results of the cognitive-behavioral intervention versus the nondirective intervention in the Kirkley and colleagues study,[245] the full versus brief intervention in the Ordman and Kirshenbaum study,[344] and the addition of exposure and response prevention to cognitive restructuring in the study by Wilson and colleagues.[475]

Fairburn and colleagues' study[106] is in some ways surprising in that a full intervention that did not directly address eating symptoms but instead focused on interpersonal issues was as effective as CBT, raising the very important point that other forms of structured psychotherapy that do not directly address eating behavior may succeed with these patients. This finding runs counter to the current treatment practices in most research

Table 24. Involvement, Completion, and Outcomes in Controlled Treatment Studies

Author(s)	Method	Started	Did Not Complete	Completed	Reduced Frequency[a] of Binge-Eating Pre-to Post-Tx	Abstinent Last Week of Tx
		Group				
Connors et al.	Psychoeducational	26	6 (23%)	20 (77%)	58%	
Yates & Sambrailo	CBT + Behavioral	24	8 (33%)	8 (? %)		1 (13%)
	CBT			8 (? %)		0 (0%)
Kirkley et al.	CBT	14	1 (7%)	13 (93%)	97%	
	Nondirective	14	5 (36%)	9 (64%)	64%	
Lee & Rush	CBT	15	4 (27%)	11 (73%)	70%	4 (29%)
Wilson et al.	Cog. restruct. + ERP	9	3 (33%)	6 (67%)	82%	5 (71%)
	Cog. restruct.	8	2 (25%)	6 (75%)	51%	2 (33%)
Leitenberg	CBT + ERP (ms)	13	1 (8%)	12 (92%)	67%*	5 (42%)
	CBT + ERP (ss)	13	2 (15%)	11 (85%)	73%*	4 (36%)
	CBT	12	0 (0%)	12 (100%)	40%*	1 (8%)

[a] Mean reduction in frequency of binge-eating
CBT—cognitive-behavioral therapy
Cog. restruct.—cognitive restructuring
ERP—exposure/response prevention
ms—multiple settings
ss—single setting

Table 24. (continued)

Author(s)	Method	Started	Did Not Complete	Completed	Reduced Frequency[a] of Binge-Eating Pre-to Post-Tx	Abstinent Last Week of Tx
		Individual				
Ordman & Kirschenbaum	Full	10	0 (0%)	10 (100%)	79%	2 (20%)
	Brief	10	0 (0%)	10 (100%)	29%	2 (20%)
Fairburn	CBT	12	1 (8%)	11 (92%)	87%	3 (27%)
	Short-term focal	12	1 (8%)	11 (92%)	82%	4 (36%)
		Mixed				
Lacey	Individual + group	30	0 (0%)	30 (100%)	95%	24 (80%)
Freeman et al.	CBT	40	14 (35%)	26 (65%)	94%	
	Behavioral Therapy				92%	
	Group				93%	
Wolchik et al.	Individual + group	13	2 (15%)	11 (85%)	58%	1 (9%)
Mitchell et al.	Group CBT + imipramine	99	19 (19%)	80 (81%)	90%	
	Group CBT + placebo				90%	
	Imipramine				70%	
	Placebo				26%	

[a] Mean reduction in frequency of binge-eating
CBT – cognitive-behavioral therapy
Cog. restruct. – cognitive restructuring
ERP – exposure/response prevention
ms – multiple settings
ss – single setting

Table 25. Follow-up Results in Controlled Treatment Studies

Author(s)	Method	Duration	Total N	N Lost	N Reduced Symptoms[a]	Abstinent at Follow-up
		Group				
Connors et al.	Psychoeducational	10 wks.	20	0 (0%)	11 (55%)	3 (15%)
Yates & Sambrailo	CBT + Behavioral	6 wks.	16	0 (0%)	4 (50%)	2 (25%)
	CBT				4 (50%)	0 (0%)
Kirkley et al.	CBT	3 mos.	22	0 (0%)	10 (76%)[b]	5 (38%)
	Non-directive				7 (78%)	1 (11%)
Lee & Rush	CBT	3–4 mos.	14	0 (0%)	7 (36%)	2 (14%)
Wilson et al.	Cog. restruct. + ERP	6 mos.	10	2 (20%)	5 (83%)	3 (50%)
	Cog. restruct.				3 (75%)	1 (25%)
Leitenberg et al.	CBT + ERP (ms)	6 mos.	10	2 (17%)	9 (90%)[c]	5 (50%)
	CBT + ERP (ss)		11	0 (0%)	8 (73%)	2 (18%)
	CBT		12	0 (0%)	8 (67%)	4 (33%)

[a]Number of patients who had reduced binge-eating frequency by >50% at follow-up
[b]Number who had reduced binge-eating frequency by >60% at follow-up
[c]Number who had reduced vomiting frequency by >50% at follow-up
CBT – cognitive-behavioral therapy
Cog. restruct. – cognitive restructuring
ERP – exposure/response prevention
ms – multiple settings
ss – single setting

Table 25. (continued)

Author(s)	Method	Duration	Total N	N Lost	N Reduced Symptoms[a]	Abstinent at Follow-up
Individual						
Ordman & Kirschenbaum	Full Brief					
Fairburn	CBT Short-term focal	6 mos.	22	0 (0%)		6 (55%) 6 (55%)
Mixed						
Lacey	Individual + group	"up to 2 yr."	29	0 (0%)	28 (97%)	20 (69%)
Freeman et al.	CBT Behavior therapy Group					
Wolchik et al.	Individual + group	10 wks.	11	0 (0%)	7 (64%)	1 (9%)

[a]Number of patients who had reduced binge-eating frequency by >50% at follow-up
[b]Number who had reduced binge-eating frequency by >60% at follow-up
[c]Number who had reduced vomiting frequency by >50% at follow-up
CBT – cognitive-behavioral therapy
Cog. restruct. – cognitive restructuring
ERP – exposure/response prevention
ms – multiple settings
ss – single setting

Table 26. Behavioral Treatment Components in the Controlled Psychotherapy Trials

Author(s)	Methods	Behavioral Components					
		Self-Monitor	Cognit. Rest.	Cue Restric.	Alter. Behav.	Delay Vomit	ERP
	Group Therapy						
Connors et al.	Psychoeducational	+	+		+		
Yates & Sambrailo	CBT + behavioral	+	+		+	+	
	CBT	+	+	+			
Kirkley et al.	CBT	+	+	+	+	+	
	Nondirective	+		+			
Lee & Rush	CBT	+	+		+		
Wilson et al.	Cog. restruct. + ERP	+	+				+
	Cog. restruct.	+	+				
Leitenberg et al.	CBT + ERP (ms)	+	+		+	+	+
	CBT + ERP (ss)	+	+		+	+	+
	CBT	+	+		+	+	

CBT—cognitive-behavioral therapy
Cog. restruct.—cognitive restructuring
ERP—exposure/response prevention
ms—multiple settings
ss—single setting

Table 26. (continued)

Author(s)	Methods	Behavioral Components					
		Self-Monitor	Cognit. Rest.	Cue Restric.	Alter. Behav.	Delay Vomit	ERP
Individual							
Ordman & Kirschen-baum	Full	+	+				+
	Brief	+			+	+	
Fairburn	CBT	+	+	+	+		
	Short-term focal	+			+		
Mixed							
Lacey	Individual + group	+	+				
Freeman et al.	CBT	+	+				
	Behavioral Therapy Group	+					
Wolchik et al.	Individual + group	+	+	+	+		
Mitchell et al.	Group CBT + im-ipramine	+	+	+	+	+	
	Group CBT + placebo Imipramine	+	+	+		+	+

CBT—cognitive-behavioral therapy
Cog. restruct.—cognitive restructuring
ERP—exposure/response prevention
ms—multiple settings
ss—single setting

Table 27. Nutritional and Other Approaches to the Controlled Psychotherapy Trials

Author(s)	Methods	Nutritional				Other	
		Modify Eat Pattern	Nutr. Educ.	Meal Plan	Reint. Feared Foods	Assert. Train.	Relax. Train.
	Group Therapy						
Connors et al.	*Psychoeducational*	+					
Yates & Sambrailo	CBT + Behavioral	+				+	+
	CBT					+	+
Kirkley et al.	CBT	+	+	+	+	+	+
	Nondirective						
Lee & Rush	CBT	+		+			
Wilson et al.	Cog. restruct. + ERP	+					+
	Cog. restruct.	+					
Leitenberg et al.	CBT + ERP (ms)	+			+		
	CBT + ERP (ss)	+			+		
	CBT	+			+		

CBT—cognitive-behavioral therapy
Cog. restruct.—cognitive restructuring
ERP—exposure/response prevention
ms—multiple settings
ss—single setting

Table 27. (continued)

Author(s)	Methods	Nutritional				Other	
		Modify Eat Pattern	Nutr. Educ.	Meal Plan	Reint. Feared Foods	Assert. Train.	Relax. Train.
Individual							
Ordman & Kirschenbaum	Full	+					
	Brief			+			
Fairburn	CBT	+					
	Short-term focal			+	+		+
Mixed							
Lacey	Individual + group	+		+			
Freeman et al.	CBT	+					
	Behavioral Therapy Group			+		+	+
Wolchik et al.	Individual + group		+	+		+	+
Mitchell et al.	Group CBT + imipramine	+	+	+	+	+	+
	Group CBT + placebo	+	+	+	+	+	+
	Imipramine	+					

CBT — cognitive-behavioral therapy
Cog. restruct. — cognitive restructuring
ERP — exposure/response prevention
ms — multiple settings
ss — single setting

centers, where researchers are specifically devising programs designed to address the eating and weight problems of patients with bulimia nervosa. This deserves further study.

The single theoretical and clinical thread running through most of the published treatment literature is the use of cognitive restructuring and behavioral techniques. The actual therapeutic variables mentioned in these programs are summarized in tables 26 and 27. First, I have grouped together behavioral components. All of the structured programs reported have used self-monitoring techniques, and most authors assume, quite rightly I believe, that the simple act of self-monitoring will improve eating behavior; therefore, this strategy is highly recommended. Whether or not to weigh patients and whether or not to use a formal treatment contract with each patient is more variable. All the published studies have included cognitive restructuring, although only a few have provided details as to how this is accomplished. In general, this involves getting the patient to examine her own cognitions, beliefs, and underlying assumptions around her eating behavior, weight, and shape.

Several programs emphasize cue restriction, such as avoiding situations, foods, or other cues that might precipitate binge-eating early in therapy; and several programs specifically include a provision encouraging patients to develop a repertoire of alternative behaviors, such as generating a list of things they can do at the times when they are most likely to binge-eat or are feeling the urge to binge-eat. A few programs ask patients to delay vomiting after binge-eating in an attempt to dissociate the binge-eating from the reinforcing vomiting response. Techniques of exposure and response prevention (ERP) are employed by several programs. Rosen, Leitenberg, and colleagues[267,268,385,386] have written persuasively in this area, having employed ERP as a primary treatment modality, wherein patients were asked to eat, and at times overeat or binge-eat, but were then prevented from the vomiting response. This has also been incorporated into the work of Wilson and colleagues. Our program uses a somewhat different but related approach. First, all patients eat dinner with the therapists on a regular basis during the course of treatment, and eventually structure into their meals the use of feared/forbidden foods and episodes of overeating.

Most programs include a nutritional counseling component (table 27), and again many authors strongly support this as a useful strategy. The content and logistics of this component vary a great deal among programs, from the simple directive for patients to try to eat regular balanced meals to the use of structured meal-planning techniques, sometimes codified in manuals. In general, there is a strong emphasis on getting patients to modify their eating patterns, not just by decreasing their bulimic behavior but also by beginning to eat regular balanced meals. Some programs specifically discuss the necessity to have patients reintroduce "feared" foods, and foods they have avoided eating because these foods are "triggers" for binge-eating episodes.

Some programs also mention assertiveness training and relaxation training.

Based on this review, we can conclude the following points about the published psychotherapy treatment studies:

1. All but one of the published controlled studies that employed two or more active treatments used programs that specifically focused on changing eating behavior. The results of the Fairburn and colleagues study,[100] using a treatment method (short-term focal therapy) that did not directly address eating patterns, but instead focused on interpersonal issues, were surprising and suggest that other types of interventions may also be effective. However the weight of the literature clearly suggests efficacy for structured programs that use specific techniques to alter eating behavior.

2. Self-monitoring is widely utilized and should be considered a very important part of treatment.

3. Cognitive behavioral techniques, to be discussed in more detail, have received a great deal of emphasis in this literature and are considered one of the most important elements in treatment by many authors, including me.

4. The one psychotherapy-versus-drug comparison study suggests that a structured intensive CBT group approach is superior to drug treatment alone in the treatment of bulimic outpatients, but the final results of this study have yet to be published.[314]

5. There are significant differences, both in terms of content (e.g., specific techniques employed) and process issues (e.g., the duration of treatment, frequency of visits, duration of visits) among the published studies.

Clearly there are many important questions yet to be answered. We really don't know about long-term outcome for most of these treatment programs, and longer-term, larger follow-up studies are indicated.

There are other logistical questions. Should there be a clear expectation of the interruption of bulimic behaviors early in treatment? Does the persistence of bulimic behavior at the end of treatment, even at low frequency, indicate a risk for relapse, or should this be viewed as the natural course of improvement and not necessarily indicative of a poor outcome? Which patients will do best with which type of treatment? Which patients would do better with drug therapy? Clearly, much has to be done; however, clinicians working in the field can learn a great deal from what has been published. In the next chapter we will focus on the details of some of the methodologies that seem to me most valuable and offer suggestions for their implementation.

10

Treatment Techniques

In this chapter I will comment on strategies that can be used in the treatment of patients with bulimia nervosa, and offer several specific techniques. In general, these techniques can be used in both individual and group therapy, and in both inpatient and outpatient settings.

The primary strategy I will outline is highly structured, and utilizes psychoeducational, behavioral, and cognitive-behavioral techniques, as well as the nutritional counseling techniques discussed previously. The major goal of this strategy is to provide patients with the skills and knowledge they need to gain control of their bulimic behaviors and to replace them with healthier, more adaptive habits. Some therapists may wish to use a few of these techniques, but to rely primarily on other strategies. I urge caution with such an approach. Certain therapeutic techniques do not mix well. My own sense is that behavioral/cognitive-behavioral therapy is most effective when it is consistently applied, highly structured, and follows logically step by step. If the patient knows that she will be following a set program, her cooperation, her compliance with the homework, and the likelihood that she will earnestly try to use the tools provided will be enhanced. These techniques demand that the therapist be active, and at times directive; therefore, they do not synthesize well with insight-oriented and/or psychodynamic therapies in which therapists are mainly nondirective and interpretive. To integrate both approaches, therapists would need to alternate roles so dramatically as to confuse both the patient and themselves.

There are certain requisites in using a highly structured approach. First, the patient must have some motivation to change her behavior. Second, she must have the necessary time and energy to devote to therapy, since such a program requires a great deal of both. Third, there can be no more pressing problem demanding the therapist's attention, such as severe depression, severe personality disorder with acting out behavior, or organic impairment. This program requires that other issues be either relatively unimportant, or at least not so severe that they cannot wait for attention. However, the strategy can be employed as part of a treatment sequence; for example, a therapist might choose to work on personality issues with a patient who has a personality disorder, and then to use the following strategy to address the eating problems.

Many of the techniques I will discuss incorporate or derive from the work of Garner, Bemis, and Fairburn, who pioneered the use of CBT in eating disorders and whose writings have been very influential in the development of psychotherapy strategies for these patients.[95,96,97,98,100,101, 103,106,121,122 125] Ferguson's work on the behavioral treatment of obesity also has been important in the development of this approach,[109] as has that of Bruch, who was an early advocate for an active therapy approach with eating disorder patients.[47]

Many of the following techniques are included in individual and group psychotherapy treatment manuals used in the University of Minnesota Eating Disorders Program. Copies of these manuals are available at cost by writing the Eating Disorders Program, University of Minnesota, Department of Psychiatry, Box 393, University of Minnesota Hospital and Clinic, 400 Delaware St. S.E., Minneapolis, MN 55455.

In undertaking such a structured approach, the first step is to prepare the individual for the therapy by establishing certain ground rules. It is wise to stress that the program will be structured, that there will be a considerable amount of homework, and that the responsibility for change will rest with the patient. It is useful to tell patients that their body weight will be periodically monitored during treatment and that, with certain exceptions to be discussed later, they need to maintain their current weight. Also, the therapist should check to make sure that the proper screening, laboratory work, and physical examination have been completed. In preparing a group, the therapist should carefully educate members about confidentiality.

We turn now to several specific components and logistical considerations. First is the issue of group dining. It is useful for individuals with bulimia nervosa to eat several meals together as part of their therapy. Eating together desensitizes the patients to eating with others, allows them to practice the meal-planning techniques that they are learning, and permits the therapist an opportunity to assess each patient's meal-planning knowledge and skills. Also, group dining provides exposure and response prevention: patients are exposed to foods in amounts that may have precipitated binge-eating and/or vomiting previously, but the presence of others prevents that usual response. This is relatively easy to do with a group, in that the therapist can take the group to dinner together. Therapists who see patients individually may bring several individuals together for a group dinner. At Minnesota, we usually eat in a separate dining room in the hospital cafeteria, but in some of our groups patients and therapists go to restaurants in the area.

Second, the timing of sessions is important. While in traditional psychotherapy, therapists meet with patients a set number of times each week, usually once a week, this may not be an optimal approach in the treatment of bulimia nervosa. More intensive involvement early in the course of treatment may provide patients with the support and encouragement necessary to interrupt their pattern of behavior: visits may be scheduled less frequently after behavioral control has been established. One schedule used in our clinic involves the therapist meeting with patients in a group twice a week for two weeks in order to introduce them to the cognitive behavioral concepts they will be using, to teach them meal-planning techniques, and to have them examine the pros and cons of giving up the bulimic behavior. Patients then enter an intensive phase, wherein they attend the clinic for three hours each evening five times a week for one week and then attend on a gradually decreasing schedule after they have gained some control of their symptoms. I find such an approach very useful, although there are no data as to whether or not such a concentrated schedule early in treatment provides a better outcome. It is certainly time consuming for both therapists and patients and logistically difficult for many therapists to arrange.

Third, the time of day when treatment is held is also important. Many patients binge-eat in the evening, and therapy scheduled then provides a healthy alternative to bulimic behavior and helps to interrupt the usual pattern. However, this again places a considerable burden on therapists.

We turn now to the formal content of this approach. The rest of this chapter is divided into "units" that represent portions of material to be covered in separate therapy sessions. The following format presupposes that patients have been evaluated and are interested in psychotherapy for their problem.

Therapists may wish to use only some of these units and/or to alter the sequence, but I would suggest that alterations in placement be done only after careful consideration, since much of the material builds on what has come before. Although the units are presented for a group format, they are also applicable to individual therapy.

I. Unit 1: Introduction

You (the therapist) first provide the patients with an overview of the proposed treatment program and introduce behavioral/cognitive-behavioral constructs as a way of conceptualizing bulimia nervosa and the treatment approach to be used.

A. Delineate the pattern of binge-eating, purging, and fasting that characterizes bulimia nervosa; review the positive and negative aspects of the behavior; and solicit comments from group members. Positives may include the sense of mastery over weight and food intake and the feeling of relaxation, stress reduction, or altered consciousness that follows vomiting. Negatives may include the physical problems that may develop as a consequence of the disorder, as well as the depression, the sense of lack of control, and the social impairment (school problems, work problems, relationship problems) that commonly develop.

B. Illustrate the feelings or affects (e.g., depression, anxiety) and behaviors (e.g., vomiting; laxative use; diuretic and diet pill use; rumination; fasting) associated with bulimia nervosa by soliciting these items from patients. Encourage the patients to begin linking these maladaptive feelings and behaviors to specific thoughts and misconceptions, such as those concerning food, weight, and self-worth. What thoughts seem to precipitate binge-eating? Vomiting? What thoughts do the patients have about their weight and eating? (e.g., "I feel fat, so I'll skip breakfast.")

C. Discuss with the patients how people with bulimia nervosa repeatedly struggle to overcome the problem. Therefore, all or most of the patients in group will have failed repeatedly in their attempts to stop. ("I'll quit tomorrow.") Point out that their past failures do not mean that they cannot learn to control the behavior. It is important to stress that things can change, because an enhanced sense of self-efficiency may improve outcome.[397]

D. Stress that improvement is not always continuous during the process of recovery. Individuals frequently have emotional ups and downs, and may have "slips," even if they temporarily gain control of their eating; but these slips can serve as important learning experiences.

E. Explain the rationale and goal of the treatment. The main goal is to replace bulimic behaviors with a healthy eating pattern, not just to stop binge-eating and vomiting. This will be accomplished by using behavioral techniques to interrupt the binge-purge cycle, and examining and understanding one's cognitions or thoughts as a way of controlling emotions and behaviors.

F. It is useful to draw up a schedule of the program with the patients and provide them with a copy.

G. As homework, instruct patients to keep complete food records and to self-monitor bulimic symptoms until they return. Tell them that the records will be reviewed and used during the next visit. (An example of a food record form is shown in figure 3, p. 68.) This form encourages patients to begin linking thoughts and feelings to their eating behavior. Also ask them to record bulimic symptoms, using a form like the one shown in figure 5. Many patients will have avoided thinking about the extent of their eating problems prior to treatment. Self-monitoring brings the problems into better focus, and many patients will be surprised by the severity of their symptoms.

H. If patients are using laxatives for weight control, it is important to address this behavior early in treatment. There are several specific issues to discuss:

1. Although most patients who abuse laxatives to control weight, think they are preventing the absorption of food and thus avoiding weight gain, in reality they are causing themselves to lose large amounts of fluid and electrolytes in the diarrhea. They may feel thinner after taking laxatives, but actually they are dehydrated, and their bodies will retain fluid in response to this, making them weigh more and feel edematous the next day. In summary, people who repeatedly use laxatives for weight control are inducing alternating states of dehydration and overhydration, not changing body fat.

2. Many patients do not understand the differences among laxatives. The ones abused by eating disorder patients are the stimulant-type laxatives such as ExLax® amd Correctol®, while some laxatives, such as Metamucil®, can be safe and useful in the treatment of constipation, including the rebound constipation encountered when discontinuing stimulant laxatives. Patients also need to be educated about the possible

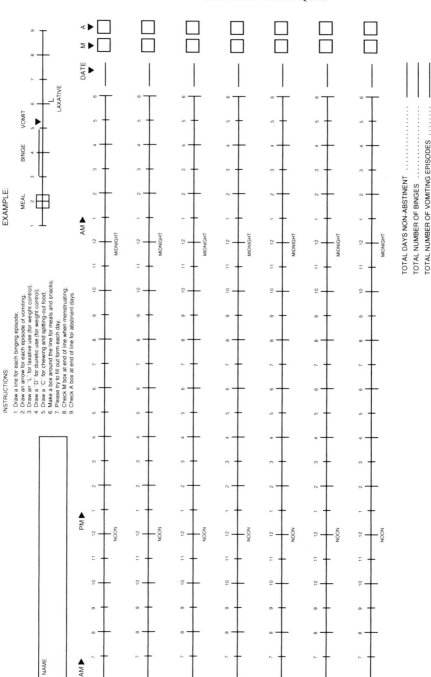

Figure 5. Eating Behaviors III Form to Record Bulimic Behaviors

consequences of laxative abuse, including dehydration, electrolyte abnormalities, and reflex fluid retention, as well as GI bleeding, bowel dysfunction, and the loss of protein in the stools. These problems are discussed in more detail in chapter 5.

3. Instruct patients in the proper way to discontinue the laxative.

a. Discontinue all stimulant-type laxatives immediately; tapering only prolongs the agony.

b. Drink a minimum of 6 to 10 cups of water or decaffeinated beverage a day. Restricting fluid intake to prevent the reflex fluid retention is not helpful and may worsen constipation, although sodium restriction may be useful. Don't add salt to food.

c. Exercise, within reasonable limits, is a way to stimulate bowel function.

d. Add bulk to the diet, e.g., eat raw fruit, to improve bowel functioning.

e. Monitor stools, and if you do not have bowel movements every three to four days, consult the therapist.

Of particular importance, bulimic patients need to be educated in detail about the temporary fluid retention that will likely result when they discontinue laxatives. They should be told that they may gain as much as 2 to 5 kgs, but that this fluid retention stops, usually in 10 to 14 days. Some temporary fluid retention is unavoidable in most cases. The rest of the session can be devoted to working on nutritional issues, in particular learning meal planning skills, as outlined in the previous chapter.

II. Unit 2: Meal Planning

A. As in all sessions, review the homework from the previous session and discuss any problems in completing it. Review the eating records with the patients, and assess their patterns of food intake and bulimic symptoms. Ask the patients what they perceive as the deficiencies in their food intake patterns and whether or not their eating patterns, as self-monitored, were surprising to them. What did they learn from the exercise?

B. The session can include a discussion of what the patients can expect as they attempt to change their eating behaviors, including the following:

1. Physiological changes are frequent; not uncommonly patients will notice gas, abdominal pain, and bloating when they first start to eat regular, balanced meals. Part of this may relate to the delayed gastric emptying that develops when people are actively bulimic. Part of this

results from a feeling of fullness, which many bulimic patients perceive as uncomfortable.

2. Unpleasant thoughts and feelings that were supressed while binge-eating may surface. Some individuals notice that when they are no longer binge-eating and vomiting that they feel demoralized, depressed, overemotional, irritable, or angry. Encourage them to bring these feelings to the group.

3. Reassure patients that whenever anyone is faced with something new, they experience some anxiety and concern about what will happen. The meal-planning techniques they are being taught initially seem confusing to some patients and can cause much anxiety. Reassure them that you will be available to answer their questions and that if they persevere, they will soon master the techniques and find them useful.

C. Instruct subjects further in the meal-planning system. Ask them to write a meal plan for the next day's meals and to repeat this task each day during the early part of treatment. They should set aside 10 to 30 minutes (but no more than 30 minutes) each day to make the meal plan. After the evening meal or before bed is a good time to do this. Above all, the meal plan should be practical. Patients should make every effort to eat what is on the meal plan each day. Make clear that the purpose of the meal-planning system is to train or retrain them in what and when they should be eating, and that initially they should eat what is on their meal plan, regardless of what they feel like eating. Instruct them not to use internal (e.g., hunger) or external (e.g., what food they encounter) cues for food choice or time of eating; such cues may be unreliable because of the bulimia nervosa. They will be able to use such cues again when they have reestablished a normal pattern.

III. Unit 3: Identifying Bulimic Behavior

A. Review homework from unit 2, including meal plans. Again, the homework review should be standard in each session, although I will not repeat this in each unit. Ask patients to continue the meal-planning techniques during the earlier part of treatment and assure them that they will find them increasingly easy to complete.

B. It is useful at this point to make sure that the patients all have a clear sense of their specific bulimic behaviors. Some behaviors are obviously pathological to most patients; most know that binge-eating and self-induced vomiting or laxative abuse are problems. However, patients might not label other practices, such as using over-the-counter diuretics, drinking large amounts of caffeine-containing liquids, restrictive eating and dieting, fasting, and excessive, inappropriate exercise for weight loss as problem behaviors.

C. Again, strongly emphasize eating all the food on the meal plan, as it is written. In most groups, there is considerable resistance to this initially. Following are some common reasons/excuses:

    1. "I've never been able to eat breakfast."

    2. "You don't understand, I'm different. If I eat this much food I'll gain weight."

    3. "I've never liked meat."

    4. "I have food allergies."

You must tell patients firmly that it is in their best interests to follow a balanced meal plan, to eat three meals a day, and to strive for variety. If they gain weight other than fluid weight, the plan can be altered, but first they should try it. Given a therapist who is firm about this, most patients will be willing to try to eat regular balanced meals. I think this is easier to accomplish in a group, since the more mature and accessible patients will exert pressure on the others to "at least try."

D. Discuss the reasons for and against (pro and con) bulimic eating habits. It is useful to have patients make lists, with reasons for stopping in one column, and reasons against stopping in the other. This can be part of the homework for the next session.

IV. Unit 4: Committment to Change

A. Discuss the pros and cons concerning ceasing or continuing bulimic behaviors. Most patients will list far more reasons to quit than not to quit, though rarely you will encounter a patient who has decided at this point not to quit. In the process of making the list, most patients realize that they are to some extent ambivalent about stopping, but that their desire to quit is stronger than their desire to continue. It is useful to recognize this ambivalence, and indicate that it does not prevent recovery.

B. Introduce the patients to the concept of alternative behaviors. Explain that they need to develop a list of alternative behaviors to replace binge-eating/vomiting. Some should be short-term behaviors that can be instituted quickly when they are faced with a desire to binge-eat, such as brushing their teeth or walking around the block. Others should be longer term, such as planning alternative activities for Saturday night if that is a prime binge-eating time. It is useful to give patients a list, like the one that follows, to which they can add items:

1. Call another group member or a friend, keep calling until you reach someone.

2. Write out the binge-eating episode rather than doing it.

3. Take a bath or shower.

4. Take a walk.

5. Watch a TV program.

6. Go to a movie.

Above all, the items should be practical.

C. At this point most patients are fairly knowledgeable and skillful in using meal-planning techniques, have examined whether or not they wish to improve their behavior, and are starting to develop a repertoire of behavioral alternatives. You can now shift to a more intensive model, if such an approach is to be used, and if the patients have been properly prepared.

Patients may verbally contract to attempt to eat regular balanced meals and cease bulimic behaviors. Some therapists prefer to use a contract in which patients attempt to gradually decrease the frequencies of these behaviors. I prefer an attempt at complete interruption, but must stress that this be done with great care. It is important not to contribute to a sense of failure in the patient. If the patient decides to try to interrupt the bulimic behaviors, it must also be made clear that many individuals who attempt this will have episodes of symptoms (slips or lapses) and that these should be regarded as an opportunity to understand the situations, feelings, and thoughts responsible for the symptoms, rather than evidence of failure or relapse. If such a strategy is to be pursued, you may choose to meet with the patients three, four, or even five times a week for the next few weeks to provide for the necessary support and structure. During this time, a different unit can be covered each evening.

V. Unit 5: Overview of Bulimia Nervosa

A. Verbally reinforce success in avoiding bulimic symptoms, but do not impart a sense of guilt or shame to those who have been unsuccessful. What worked for successful patients? What can the others try differently?

B. This is a good point in treatment to make sure that patients are well educated about bulimia nervosa and about the treatment approach you are using. How do the patients see the process as going? Most patients will be more willing to ask questions several sessions into the treatment.

C. As a major focus of the session, discuss factors that are involved in the development of bulimia nervosa.

As usual, it is useful to begin by soliciting the patients' own perceptions. Usually members of a group will offer particular factors in their lives that they see as causal in the development of their eating problems, and these can be discussed for their relevance to other group members. If the following issues do not emerge as part of the discussion, introduce them and have group members discuss them:

1. Bulimia nervosa is strongly linked to cultural factors, in that the disorder appears almost exclusively in societies where there is a marked emphasis on thinness and having a youthful appearance. In what ways is this cultural bias reinforced? Discussion can include advertising on television and in the print media.

2. I find it useful to present information about the regulation of body weight, and I use set-point theory as a model to illustrate the biology of weight regulation. I review briefly animal research that suggests that body weight is regulated by the hypothalamus and other centers in the brain. I also briefly review studies in humans that indicate a strong genetic component in adult body weight. I then tie this to the problem of eating disorders, suggesting that individuals who are always trying to be too thin may be fighting their own physiology or programmed set-weight range, and that this has undesirable consequences. The notion that people have a biologically programmed set-point to which their bodies naturally tend to gravitate is a surprising, often initially upsetting idea for some patients, but as they come to realize the implications of the concept it can be quite helpful therapeutically.

3. Review metabolic changes that result from bulimia nervosa, in particular the fact that metabolic efficiency changes in an undesirable direction—that patients tend to gain weight on less food intake while actively bulimic. This is a particularly powerful argument for gaining control of binge-eating and vomiting and eating regularly.

VI. Unit 6: Cues and Consequences

A. Review the progress on interruption of bulimic behaviors. As before, improvement should be verbally reinforced. What worked for the successful patients? Assess episodes of bulimic symptoms, with the goal of identifying specific cues that triggered the episodes and the development of suitable, practical behavioral alternatives.

B. The main thrust of this unit is to begin to addressing in detail the cues and consequences associated with bulimic symptoms. It is important to carefully explain the concept of cues and consequences.

The word *cue* can be defined as the events that occur before a response.

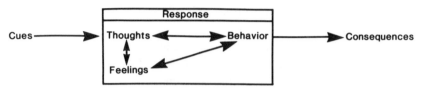

Figure 6. The Relationships among Cues, Responses (Thoughts, Feelings, Behaviors),
and Consequences

Responses can be thoughts, feelings, or behaviors; they are caused, or cued, by what happens before them. A response is encouraged or discouraged by consequences—events that occur after the response. Cues and consequences are illustrated in figure 6.

Many sorts of cues may be involved in triggering bulimic behavior. These may be social (e.g. attending a family dinner), situational (e.g., advertisements depicting very thin women, eating 'forbidden foods'), physiological/nutritional (e.g., hunger, fatigue), and mental (e.g., upsetting memories, a mental image of oneself as overweight).

Both negative and positive consequences may result from bulimic behaviors. For example, some social consequences of bulimic behavior are positive (e.g., avoidance of interpersonal conflict, social reinforcement for not gaining weight), while others are negative (e.g., social isolation, lying to others, and not being trusted). Some situational consequences of bulimia nervosa are positive for some people (e.g. avoiding responsibility, avoiding independence), and some are negative (e.g., financial or work problems). Some feeling consequences are positive (e.g., relief of tension, anger, or boredom), while others are negative (e.g., depression, guilt, shame). Some thought consequences are positive (e.g., thoughts about avoiding weight gain), while others are negative (e.g. increase in guilt). Some physiological/nutritional consequences are positive (e.g. reduced hunger during and after a binge-eating episode), while others are negative (e.g., weakness, dizziness, poor concentration, dental problems).

Therefore, bulimic behavior can be conceptualized, and presented to the patient, as continuing over time because the positive consequences are more immediate than the negative consequences. It is very important for the patient to understand that, in the long run, the negative consequences are more important, although they are less immediate and therefore less closely tied to the response in her mind. There are reasons to be bulimic, but if one really understands the consequences – all the consequences – the behavior is highly undesirable.

C. In this unit you can begin to focus specifically on cues. One way to improve eating habits is to identify and learn to change or control the cues that lead to bulimic symptoms by breaking the relationship between the cue and the response. This can be done in several ways.

1. Rearrange the cues.

a. Avoidance. A simple method of rearranging cues is to avoid them. Don't walk or drive by the bakery on the way to work; avoid "trigger" foods early in treatment.

b. Restrict the stimulus field – the cues that trigger the behavior. For example, eat only at the table and don't do other things while eating. Stay away from cues that trigger binge-eating, such as watching television or reading advertisements in magazines while eating.

c. Strengthen cues for desired behaviors. Expose yourself to existing cues that lead to healthy behavior. For example, if you binge-eat at home while studying, but never while studying at the library, you should always study in the library.

2. Change your response to cues.

a. Build in a pause – delay the response. This allows you to pass through the period of highest risk, and breaks the cue from the automatic behavioral response. For example, pause for at least 15 minutes when deciding whether or not to binge-eat.

b. Choose alternative behaviors. Replace a maladaptive behavior with a competing adaptive behavior. When a cue starts to trigger an episode of binge-eating, go for a walk, call a friend, or brush your teeth.

c. Exposure and response prevention. Make bulimic behavior after eating a meal unlikely or impossible. For example, take no extra money to work so there won't be money for candy from the snack machines after you eat lunch; eat only with your family and friends and never alone; take a walk after you eat with a friend. In this way you expose yourself to food and to eating, but prevent a vomiting response.

It is also helpful to rearrange the consequences of behavior, so that appropriate behaviors will be rewarded, and inappropriate behaviors not rewarded. Certain guidelines can be offered in terms of rewards. First, the reward should follow rather than precede the behavior, and the reward should be contingent on the occurrence of the behavior. No behavior, no reward. Second, the reward should follow the behavior as quickly as possible.

There are two types of rewards: mental (thoughts), and material or activity (things). Mental rewards are those you imagine or say to yourself, such as a compliment for something you have done well or for some characteristic, or simply imagining something pleasant. For example, "I really did a good job today," or "It took some doing but I was able to avoid stopping at the bakery," or "I am dependable." Mental rewards are useful because they can be used any time, anywhere, are tailor-made to the person and can be given immediately after she accomplishes her goal. Material or activity rewards can also be tailor-made, but usually require more planning; they might include going to a movie or play, spending time on a favorite hobby, or buying a favorite record album.

D. As a homework assignment, ask patients to work on their cues and consequences. First they should list at least three cues that are associated with their bulimic behaviors, and then consider strategies that they can use to rearrange these cues to minimize the occurrence of the behavior. They should also work on rearranging the consequences of their bulimia. For example, they can define a goal behavior that they would like to achieve and then spell out when, where, and how frequently they want to accomplish this goal. An example would be to write out the next day's meal plan and then decide on a specific reward for meeting the goal; for example, calling a friend long distance.

VII. Unit 7: Responses

A. While the previous unit focused on cues and consequences, this unit will focus on responses, the middle part of the cue-response- consequence sequence. Review the components of the sequence as outlined in Figure 7, including the three types of responses: thoughts, behaviors, and feelings. Behaviors are actions the patient takes that can be observed by others, if others are present. Thoughts and feelings are internal states and therefore private, more difficult to identify and more difficult for others to observe. Thoughts are particularly important in determining how a person reacts to a situation or cue; the thoughts a person has regarding a particular situation or cue will influence how she feels and how she behaves.

Offering the following example will prove helpful: Imagine two people passing by a bakery. One person has bulimia nervosa and the other has no significant eating problems. They may have very different reactions to the bakery. While the second person may walk past the bakery without giving it a second thought, or may stop and buy rolls or some sort of dessert, the person with bulimia nervosa may feel anxious and experience a strong urge to binge-eat. The differences in reactions are primarily due to their different thoughts regarding the bakery. The person without bulimia nervosa may think, "It would be nice to have good rolls or a dessert for after dinner. I like fresh bakery goods." The other person may think, "I haven't had anything to eat all day; I deserve something sweet; I deserve to binge-eat after a hard day. Nothing will help me relax except a binge."

People with bulimia nervosa develop lots of thoughts such as these as part of their disorder. Some are so common as to be almost ubiquitous among these patients; for example, "If I eat a regular meal, I'll get fat," and "I am too fat, I need to be thinner."

Such thoughts eventually become automatic, in the same way as one drives along a familiar route on "automatic pilot," without really remembering the trip. Likewise, people with bulimia nervosa may find that they are upset but be unaware of the thoughts that are upsetting them. As an example, have the patient imagine that she just ate an extra piece of cake — cake that was not on her meal plan. What are her thoughts associated with this situation? What are her feelings associated with this situation? How might she behave in this situation? Patients usually can identify feelings much more easily than their underlying thoughts. It is useful to go through several such examples. Many people with eating problems also have certain styles of thinking that are maladaptive and can lead to maladaptive responses. Some of those negative thinking styles are described below:

1. *Overgeneralization* — deciding on a rule based on the experience of one event and then applying it inappropriately to other situations. (Example: "Nobody likes me," "I'm never going to be able to control my eating.")

2. *Catastrophizing* — embellishing a situation with too much meaning, beyond what is supported by the evidence, thinking of things in too extreme a manner. (Examples: "I've eaten more than is on my meal plan; I'm a failure," "I'm going to be late; this is terrible.")

3. *Dichotomous thinking* — "all or nothing" thinking. (Examples: "I've had one bite too much, I might as well binge-eat," "If I gain one pound, I will continue to gain weight and get fat.")

4. *Self-fulfilling ideas*—making predictions about what will happen, then acting in such a way that the behavior ensures that outcome. (Example: "I don't know what I will do if I gain even a pound. I know I'll feel terrible," "If I feel too full, I have to vomit.")

5. *Over-reliance on the opinions of others*—(Example: "If I gain weight, I don't want to go out or be seen. Everyone will think I'm fat.") Have each patient discuss an example of each of these styles.

B. As the last part of this unit, introduce worksheets to help patients with restructuring thoughts. An example is shown as figure 7. Teach patients to identify the cues, the responses (thoughts, feelings, and behaviors), and the consequences, and ask them to complete several of these as part of their homework before returning.

VIII. Unit 8: Restructuring Thoughts

A. As the previous units focused on the first steps in restructuring thoughts that are linked to bulimic behaviors—becoming aware of the thoughts, feelings, and behaviors that are triggered by particular cues and that result in specific consequences—this unit focuses on having patients evaluate their thoughts in order to determine whether or not they are accurate and reasonable. I will discuss two methods to teach patients to challenge and determine the accuracy of their thoughts, a crucial step in the process of cognitive restructuring.

The first technique is to challenge the thoughts by questioning their content. Is the thought really accurate? What is the evidence to support or refute the thought? What are the alternative explanations (thoughts) that would substitute for the thought being examined?

Let us use an example: The cue is that the patient has eaten a chocolate chip cookie. The thoughts might be "I'm going to get fat if I don't vomit, so I might as well binge-eat." The resultant behavior might be binge-eating and vomiting, the associated feelings might be guilt and remorse, and the resulting consequences might be self-disgust, and the perpetuation of the behavior, as well as a sense of failure. Have the patient evaluate the thought. What is the evidence for the thought? Is there evidence to support the thought? Not really. To refute the thought? Yes, eating one cookie will not make anyone fat, and vomiting is not really an effective means of weight control. What are the implications of the thought? Even if the thought were true, it would not ruin the individual's life. Consideration can then be given to revising the thought. One revised thought might be that even though the patient has eaten the cookie, it is better not to binge-

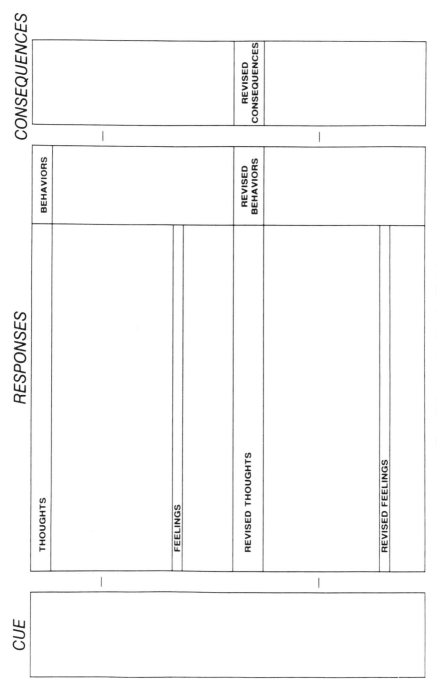

Figure 7. Restructuring Thoughts Worksheet

eat, since it will only cause depression and perpetuate the bulimic behaviors. Also, one cookie is really "no big deal," and it should not make
her feel fat or feel like a failure. Revised feelings might be a decrease in
anxiety and revised behavior might be not binge-eating and vomiting. The
revised consequences would be a sense of achievement and control.

It is useful then to review the sequence we have followed:
1. Identify the cue
2. Identify the thoughts
3. Identify the feelings
4. Identify the behaviors
5. Identify the consequences
6. Evaluate the thoughts by examining the evidence that supports the
thoughts and the evidence that refutes the thoughts, examining the implications of the thoughts, and looking at alternative thoughts. Then
consider modifying the thoughts.

A second method is to challenge maladaptive thoughts and erroneous
assumptions by testing them prospectively. The patient can be encouraged to set up experiments to test their accuracy. Suppose that a
patient believes that eating three meals a day will cause her to gain
weight and become obese, a very common thought among this group
of patients. How can she test that assumption?

B. Patients should be assigned the restructuring thoughts worksheets.

IX. Unit 9: Cues and chains

A. It is useful to review the model of cues, responses (thoughts, feelings, and behaviors), and consequences to make sure that the patients understand it.

Afterwards, you can point out that the occurrence of behavior often
cannot be explained using only these five components in one sequence. Instead, much of the time behavior consists of a series of components, each
representing one link in a long chain. For example, a cue triggers a response, which then becomes a cue itself for another set of responses, and
so on. In figure 8, an example of such a chain is demonstrated. Have patients prepare such a chain based on one of their bulimic episodes, either
a recent one or, if they are in control of their bulimic symptoms, one from
memory.

The focus then becomes an investigation of the ways that the chain can
be broken early in the cycle. The earlier the chain is broken, the easier

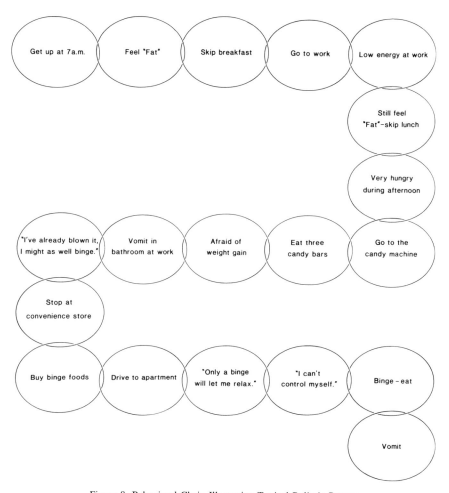

Figure 8. Behavioral Chain Illustrating Typical Bulimic Pattern

it is to prevent the occurrence of bulimic symptoms. Several strategies discussed before are useful here:

1. Rearrange cues.
    a. Avoid the cue.
    b. Eliminate the cue.
    c. Restrict the stimulus field.
    d. Strengthen cues that promote healthy behavior.
2. Change responses to cues.
    a. Build in a delay.

    b. Use alternative behaviors.

    c. Use exposure and response prevention.

  3. Rearrange the consequences — structure the rewards.

  4. Restructure thoughts.

B. For homework, have each patient complete several cues and chains, and in each sequence, indicate several places where the behavioral chain could be interrupted.

X. Unit 10: Body Image I

A. The problem of body image needs to be addressed as part of the treatment of this disorder. Though the concept has been introduced earlier in our discussion, I think it is a very important area, and that it is useful to spend a few sessions focusing on this issue. Body image can be defined as the perception or mental picture of one's physical body. Many individuals with bulimia nervosa have a distorted body image and their ideas about their own body size and shape are often inaccurate. This is not necessarily a global misperception, in that many individuals overestimate the size of only certain parts, particularly their thighs, hips, or stomach, but see other parts as being of normal size. It is useful to point out that this problem is not restricted to individuals with eating disorders and is quite common in our society at large.

There are several points that can be discussed with the patients:

  1. Do they have an accurate picture of their own body/body parts?

  2. Are they satisfied with their current weight and shape? If not, why not? What do they want to change?

  3. How much (often) do they think about their physical appearance?

  4. How important is their physical appearance to them?

  5. What are some of the messages, rules, and beliefs about their bodies or body parts that they remember learning from parents, peers, and society? (For example — "People will like you better if you are thin.")

  6. Do any of these messages or beliefs influence how they feel about their bodies today? Which ones?

  7. How can they change these beliefs/thoughts to more positive thoughts about themselves?

It is important to stress that recovery from bulimia nervosa includes becoming more accepting of one's own body, regardless of size and shape.

At this point I find it very useful to review the paper by David Garner and his colleagues concerning Miss America Pageant contestants.[125]

Table 28. Body Inventory

Please indicate on the scales below how you feel about different areas of your body.

Body Part	Very Positive	Positive	Somewhat Positive	Neutral	Somewhat Negative	Negative	Very Negative
Hair	1	2	3	4	5	6	7
Nose	1	2	3	4	5	6	7
Teeth	1	2	3	4	5	6	7
Eyes	1	2	3	4	5	6	7
Ears	1	2	3	4	5	6	7
Lips/mouth	1	2	3	4	5	6	7
Skin	1	2	3	4	5	6	7
Face	1	2	3	4	5	6	7
Arms	1	2	3	4	5	6	7
Hands	1	2	3	4	5	6	7
Breasts/chest	1	2	3	4	5	6	7
Shoulders	1	2	3	4	5	6	7
Abdomen	1	2	3	4	5	6	7
Hips	1	2	3	4	5	6	7
Back	1	2	3	4	5	6	7
Buttocks	1	2	3	4	5	6	7
Waist	1	2	3	4	5	6	7
Upper legs (thighs)	1	2	3	4	5	6	7
Lower legs (calves)	1	2	3	4	5	6	7
Feet	1	2	3	4	5	6	7
Body build	1	2	3	4	5	6	7
Posture	1	2	3	4	5	6	7

Overall how *dissatisfied* are you with the way your body is proportioned?

Extremely Dissatisfied	Very Dissatisfied	Moderately Dissatisfied	Slightly Dissatisfied	Not at All Dissatisfied
1	2	3	4	5

(Adapted with permission from the Melpomene Institute.)

They demonstrated that the average weight of the contestants in the pageant declined over the last 20 years, and that winners often weighed less than the average participant. Other issues to include are the cultural preoccupation with dieting in our society, in that 50% to 80% of girls in America have dieted by the time they reach 18.

B. For homework, have patients complete a "Body Inventory" (table 28).

XI. Unit 11: Body Image II

A. While the previous unit focused on thoughts and feelings about body size and shape, this unit focuses on patients being more accepting of their own bodies. There are several avenues through which this can be pursued. One is to have patients identify specific negative thoughts about body size and shape and attempt to challenge these thoughts using the techniques described before. This can be done in written form, using the restructuring thoughts worksheet. A second avenue is to have each patient think of her body in more functional terms. What does her body enable her to do? What does it enable her to enjoy? Even bodies that are less than "ideal" still permit a wide range of activities. At this point it is useful to have patients make a list of positive thoughts and feelings they have about their bodies, focusing on the areas that they think are their best features and on the things they enjoy that their bodies allow them to do (e.g., walk, run, play tennis). Structured in this way, most individuals will be able to identify things about their bodies about which they feel positive—perhaps their physical strength, or that they look good in a certain color clothing, or that they are a good swimmer, or that they like the shape and color of their eyes. These positive statements can be substituted as alternatives for negative thoughts about body shape and weight and can be practiced outside of the therapy. Make such a list part of the homework.

XII. Unit 12: Relapse Prevention I

A. If we assume that at this point most of the patients are in control of their eating behavior with only minor lapses, and that they are eating regular balanced meals, then you can begin to address the issue of relapse prevention. This is a particularly important area, since there is a significant potential for relapse.

It is important first to teach patients the differences between *lapses* or *slips* and *relapse*. The former are common minor recurrences of symptoms that provide an opportunity to learn and are not evidence of failure, while the latter—which entails a complete loss of control and return to the bulimic pattern—is more serious but probably preventable. This differentiation is of great importance.

B. It is useful to discuss certain rules with the patient that may help prevent relapse:

1. Attempt to keep body weight at a steady, 'normal' weight for you.
2. Don't engage in starvation, fasting, or excessive dieting.

3. Attempt to handle stress in an adaptive, functional way, and not by turning to food.

4. Practice exposure to high-risk situations and high-risk foods while in treatment. Reintroduce high-risk situations or foods that you may have excluded from your lifestyle, for if these remain "feared," they may preordain a relapse upon exposure. A good way to approach this problem is to have patients list three or four high-risk foods and high-risk situations, and then, starting with the least feared and progressing to the most feared, have them practice exposure.

Instruct patients that the time should be right; they should be sure to have the structure and support necessary so that the chances of a slip are low. For example, if an individual has avoided eating ice cream since this had been a binge food for her, she should incorporate this food back into her eating pattern. She might have a dish of ice cream at a public place with a friend who is aware of the problem. The support of the other person and the public setting will make it unlikely that she will vomit. The patient may also want to schedule a pleasurable activity immediately after eating the ice cream to combat any residual anxiety about the situation and to prevent vomiting. At the other extreme, she should not as her exposure exercise, buy ice cream and go home alone to her apartment and eat the ice cream after a long, frustrating day of work.

Assign the lowest risk food and lowest risk situation before the next visit.

XIII. Unit 13: Relapse Prevention II

A. Review the success or failure of reintroduction of a high-risk food or situation. Assign next higher risk items and have the patients decide how to reintroduce them.

B. Have patients articulate the differences between a lapse or slip and relapse. What are useful ways of dealing with a slip or lapse in order to prevent a relapse? Have the patients describe, in detail, how they would deal with a lapse of bulimic behavior after treatment.

You may also want to create a hypothetical situation. Have the patient imagine that she has successfully completed treatment and has continued in an aftercare group, but then moved away from the city in which she was treated. Five months later, she begins encountering difficulties at work and stresses in her social life. She finds it increasingly difficult to eat regular meals because of her new work schedule and becomes very concerned about her weight. She then starts skipping meals, losing weight, and eventually begins to binge-eat. Shortly thereafter she also begins self-inducing vomiting. Therefore, over a period of several weeks she has returned to a previous bulimic pattern, and is now early in the process of relapse. These questions can then be put to the patient:

1. What does she need to do about her eating behavior and meal planning?

2. What does she need to do about her vomiting?

3. What does she need to do about her thoughts concerning weight and shape?

4. What does she need to do about her social problems?

5. What are the chances that these problems will go away on their own?

C. For a homework assignment, have patients write out what they think would be the most likely scenario if they were to relapse, and how they could interrupt the pattern early in the course of the relapse. Also as a homework assignment, reintroduce another feared food/situation, again with proper controls.

XIV. Unit 14: Relapse Prevention III

A. Review homework and success or failure of exposure to high-risk situation/high-risk food.

B. Discuss the necessity for developing a healthy life-style as a means of preventing relapse. This may include the following:

1. Developing an ongoing support network, based on the individual's needs. This may include a community support group, closer ties with family, and trying to make new friends. How can these goals be met?

2. Developing a variety of healthy experiences in life that are unrelated to food or eating, such as social and leisure time activities that are rewarding, an adequate, healthy amount of exercise, and adequate time to be alone for contemplation.

C. As a homework assignment, have each patient reintroduce another high-risk food and high-risk situation, and plan the changes that she needs to make in order to develop a healthier lifestyle. Her plans should include the following elements: work, school, exercise, time alone, religion, family, friends, romantic relationships, long-term goals.

XV. Other structured components. Depending on your interests and expertise, and the needs of the individual patients, additional units can be used. Some suggestions follow:

A. An exercise unit. Some mention needs to be made of exercise in any treatment program for bulimia nervosa. However, considerable time needs to be devoted to this issue with a subgroup of patients who compulsively exercise, or those who don't exercise at all. First it is useful for individuals to quantify how much exercise they are getting in the course of their daily activities, and to discuss their purposes for exercising. Benefits of exercise may include stress reduction, improvement in mood, favorable metabolic changes, exercise as a social outlet, and exercise for a source of fun, as well as for physical fitness.

For those who need more specific guidance to begin exercising, it is useful to have them begin by walking, or engaging in some other nonstrenuous exercise, for 20 to 30 minutes, three or four times a week. Try to include at least one exercise activity a week that provides a social outlet, such as tennis or walking with a friend. Individuals should be encouraged to develop exercise habits in which availability will not be a problem (e.g., do not choose swimming if you have nowhere to swim regularly).

B. Family issues. The amount of time devoted to family issues will vary, depending on the age of the patients, whether or not they are living with their family, and whether or not family problems are uncovered. At minimum, consideration should be given to an examination of family rules and assumptions concerning food, meal times, weight, and shape. There is some evidence that patients with bulimia nervosa tend to come from families that are highly anxious about weight issues and derogatory toward overweight people.[480]

C. Stress management and problem solving. First, definitions are in order. A stressor can be defined as a demand. Stressors may be major (e.g., moving, marriage), or minor (e.g., finding a parking place, meeting a blind date). Although most people recognize and accept major stressors as potential problems, minor repetitive stressors can accumulate and take on major proportions. The patients should be instructed to attempt to recognize stressors in their lives, and to list them. Stress response is defined as the thoughts, feelings, behaviors, and physical states that are triggered by stressors. A stress cycle and stress response model can be offered (see figure 9). Using this model, patients can attempt to alter their thoughts about the stressors, and to evolve more adaptive associated behaviors and feelings, thereby influencing the consequences in positive ways.

Negative Stress Response

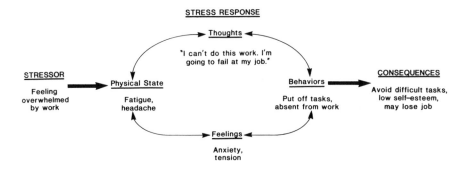

Positive Stress Response

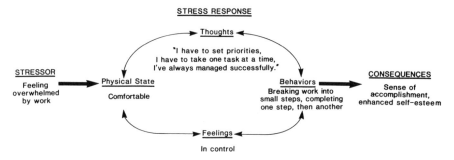

Figure 9. Stress Model Using Cognitive-Behavioral Terminology

D. Problem-solving skills can be fostered by teaching a sequence of steps:

1. Define the problem.

2. Generate a list of possible alternative solutions.

3. Evaluate each alternative.

4. Choose the one that appears to be best, knowing that the choice may be wrong, and that choices are rarely ideal.

5. Implement the choice.

6. Examine the consequences of the action. Was the proper alternative selected, or would another have been preferable in retrospect? What have you learned from the exercise? Again, concrete examples from your life will work best.

Afterword

I hope that those who read this book, or sample portions of it, find this disorder as interesting and challenging as I do. I believe there are few examples in medicine or psychology of a disorder that can have such globally adverse effects on an individual's life, yet which is clearly treatable and reversible. The other thing that I find particularly interesting about bulimia nervosa is that a number of variables must be involved in its etiology. There is growing evidence that biological, perhaps genetic, factors contribute to the risk of development of and maintenance of this disorder; second, cultural factors are important; third, psychological issues are clearly involved on either a primary or secondary basis; fourth, social functioning deteriorates; and fifth, the physiological consequences pose special management problems for mental health professionals.

Where are we going from here? It seems to me that research has progressed to a point where it is clear we have developed treatment techniques, both pharmacological and psychotherapeutic, that impact significantly on the course and outcome of this disorder. However, it is much less clear how and when these treatments should be applied. I believe considerable emphasis needs to be placed on looking at predictive variables that may anticipate the proper therapy and the proper duration of maintenance therapy for each patient.

A second area that I believe will assume increasing importance is the problem of comorbidity. As I have discussed, I do not believe bulimia nervosa can be regarded as a unique homogeneous diagnostic entity, but that it may be a manifestation of another form of psychopathology, such as alcohol/drug abuse and depression, or it may engender other psychopathology. Research on these comorbidity issues requires expertise in a variety of types of psychopathology.

A third area of particular interest is the biology of bulimia nervosa. Those involved in biological research in psychology and psychiatry are well aware that we are in the midst of a revolution in the neurosciences. Our understanding of the brain and its functioning is increasing dramatically, and I think it is safe to say that neurosciences, along with molecular biology, represent two of the "hottest" areas in research. It is only logical to assume that some of the new findings in this area will contribute to our understanding of the pathophysiology of eating problems, including bulimia nervosa.

I wish to end on an optimistic note. I recall that in the early 1980s one frequently encountered pessimism about this disorder among professionals. I think that pessimism is being replaced by an informed optimism as we begin to understand and effectively treat this disorder, and we should impart this optimism to our patients.

References

References

1. Abdu RA, Garritano D, Culver O: Acute gastric necrosis in anorexia nervosa and bulimia. Arch Surg 1987; 122:830–832

2. Abraham SF, Beumont PJV: How patients describe bulimia or binge eating. Psychol Med 1982; 12:625–635

3. Abraham SF, Buemont PJV, Cobbin DM: Catecholamine metabolism and body weight in anorexia nervosa. Br J Psychiatry 1981; 138:244–247

4. Abraham SF, Mira M, Llewellyn-Jones D: Bulimia: A study of outcome. Int J Eating Disord 1983; 2:175–180

5. Adler AO, Walinsky P, Krall RA, et al: Death resulting from ipecac syrup poisoning. JAMA 1980; 243:1927–1928

6. Agras WS, Dorian B, Kirkley BG, et al: Imipramine in the treatment of bulimia: A double-blind controlled study. Int J Eating Disord 1987; 6:29–38

7. Al-Mufty NS, Bevan DH: A case of subcutaneous emphysema, pneumomediastinum and pneumoretroperitoneum associated with functional anorexia. Br J Clin Pract 1977; 31:160–161

8. Altschuler S, Conte A, Sebok M, et al: Three controlled trials of weight loss with phenylpropanolamine. Int J Obes 1982; 6:549–556

9. Anders D, Harms D, Kriens O, et al: Zur Frage der Sialadenose als sekundarer Organmanifestation der Anorexia nervosa - Beobachtungen an einem 13 jahrigen Knaben. Klin Padiatr 1975; 187:156–162

10. Andersen AE, Mickalide AD: Anorexia nervosa and bulimia. Bull Menninger Clin 1985; 49:227–235

11. Anderson AE, Hay A: Racial and socioeconomic influences in anorexia nervosa and bulimia. Int J Eating Disord 1985; 4:479–487

12. Atkinson RL, Berke LK, Drake CR: Effects of long-term therapy with naltrexone on body weight in obesity. Clin Pharmacol Ther 1985; 38:419–422

13. Bailey RR: Water-logged women: Idiopathic oedema. NZ Med J 1977; 85:129–132

14. Barlow J, Blouin J, Blouin A, et al: Treatment of bulimia with desipramine: A double blind crossover study. Can J Psychiatry 1988; 33:129–133

15. Bartter FC, Pronove P, Gill JR, et al: Hyperplasis of the juxtaglomerular complex with hyperaldosteronism and hypokalemia alkalosis. Am J Med 1962; 33:811–828

16. Beary MD, Lacey JH, Merry J: Alcoholism and eating disorders in women of fertile age. Br J Addict 1986; 81:685–689

17. Bemis KM: "Abstinence" and "nonabstinence" models for the treatment of bulimia. Int J Eating Disord 1985; 4:407–437

149

18. Ben-Ishay D, Levy M, Birnbaum D: Self-induced secondary hyperaldosteronism simulating Bartter's syndrome. Isr J Med Sci 1972; 8:1835–1839

19. Bennett HS, Spiro AJ, Pollack MA, et al: Ipecac-induced myopathy simulating dermatomyositis. Neurology 1982; 32:91–94

20. Bennett WM: Hazards of the appetite suppressant phenylpropanolamine. Lancet 1975; 42–43

21. Bennum I: Depression and hostility in self-mutilation. Suicide Life Threat Behav 1983; 13:71–84

22. Bergen SS: Appetite-stimulating properties of cyproheptadine. Am J Dis Child 1964; 108:270–273

23. Berger BE, Warnock DG: Clinical uses and mechanisms of action of diuretic agents, in The Kidney. Edited by Brennor BM, Rector FC. Philadelphia: Saunders, 1986, pp 435–55

24. Berke GS, Calcaterra TC: Parotid hypertrophy with bulimia: A report of surgical management. Laryngoscope 1985; 95:597–598

25. Berland NW: The importance of personality assessment in the treatment of bulimia. Ala J Med Sci 1985; 22:223–224

26. Beumont PJV, George GCW, Smart DE: "Dieters" and "vomiters and purgers" in anorexia nervosa. Psychol Med 1976; 6:617–622

27. Birtchnell SA, Lacey JH, Harte A: Body image distortion in bulimia nervosa. Br J Psychiatry 1985; 147:408–412

28. Blouin AG, Blouin JH, Periz EL, et al: Treatment of bulimia with fenfluramine and desipramine. J Clin Psychopharmacol 1988; 8:261–269

29. Blouin J, Blouin A, Perez E, et al: Family history factors in bulimia. Presented at the Second International Conference on Eating Disorders, New York, April 1986

30. Bo-linn G, Santa Ana C, Morawski S, et al: Purging and calorie absorption in bulimic patients and normal women. Ann Intern Med 1983; 99:14–17

31. Boskind-Lodahl M: Cinderella's stepsisters: A feminist perspective on anorexia nervosa and bulimia. Women, Culture, and Society 1976; 2:342–356

32. Boskind-Lodahl M, White WC: The definition and treatment of bulimarexia in college women —a pilot study. J of Ach 1978; 27:84–97

33. Boskind-White M: Bulimarexia: A sociocultural perspective. In Theory and Treatment of Anorexia Nervosa and Bulimia. Edited by Emmett SW. Brunner/Mazel, Inc., New York 1985

34. Boskind-White M, White WC: Bulimiarexia: The binge/purge cycle. New York: W.W. Norton & Co., 1983

35. Breslow M, Yates A, Shisslak C: Spontaneous rupture of the stomach: A complication of bulimia. Int J Eat Dis 1986; 5:137–142

36. Brewerton TD, Brandt HA, Lesem MD, et al: Serotonin in eating disorders. In Serotonin in Major Psychiatric Disorders. Edited by Coccaro EF, Murphy DL. American Psychiatric Association Press, Washington (in press)

37. Brewerton TD, Heffernan MM, Rosenthal NE: Psychiatric aspects of the relationship between eating and mood. Nutr Rev Suppl 1986; 44:78–88

38. Brisman J, Siegel M: Bulimia and alcoholism: Two sides of the same coin? J Subst Abuse Treat 1984; 1:113–118

39. Brotman AW, Rigotti N, Herzog DB: Medical complications of eating disorders: Outpatient evaluation and management. Compr Psychiatry 1985; 26:258–271

40. Brotman MC, Forbath N, Garfinkel PE, et al: Myopathy due to ipecac syrup poisoning in a patient with anorexia nervosa. Can Med Assoc J 1981; 125:453–454

41. Brown GL, Ebert MH, Boyer PF, et al: Aggression, suicide, and serotonin: Relationships to C.S.F. amine metabolites. Am J Psychiatry 1982; 139:741–746

42. Brown NW: Medical consequences of eating disorders. South Med J 1985; 78:403–405

43. Bruch, H: Eating disorders. New York: Basic Books, 1973

44. Buckholtz NS, George DT, Davies AO, et al: Lymphocyte B-Adrenergic receptor modification in bulimia. Arch Gen Psychiatry 1988; 45:479-482

45. Bulik CA: Alcohol use and depression in women with bulimia. Am J Drug Alcohol Abuse 1987; 13:343-355

46. Bulik CM: Drug and alcohol abuse by bulimic women and their families. Am J Psychiatry 1987; 144:1604-1606

47. Bullimore DW, Cooke D: Cyclical vomiting with pneumomediastinum. Acta Paediatr Scand 1982; 71:675-676

48. Burke RC: Bulimia and parotid enlargement — Case report and treatment. J Otolaryngol 1986; 15:49-50

49. Butterfield PS, Leclair S: Cognitive characteristics of bulimic and drug- abusing women. Addict Behav 1988; 13:131-138

50. Cantwell, DP, Sturzenburger S, Burroughs J, et al: Anorexia nervosa-An affective disorder. Arch Gen Psychiatry 1977; 34:1087-1093

51. Carroll BJ: Use of the dexamethasone suppression test in depression. J Clin Psychiatry 1982; 43:44-48

52. Carroll BJ, Feinberg M, Greden JF, et al: A specific laboratory test for the diagnosis of melancholia. Arch Gen Psychiatry 1981, 38:15-22

53. Carter JA, Duncan PA: Binge-eating and vomiting: A survey of a high school population. Psychol Schools 1984; 21:198-203

54. Carter PI, Moss RA: Screening for anorexia and bulimia nervosa in a college population: Problems and limitations. Addict Behav 1984; 9:417-419

55. Casper RC, Eckert ED, Halmi, SC, et al: Bulimia: Its incidence and clinical importance in patients with anorexia nervosa. Arch Gen Psychiatry 1980; 37:1036-1040

56. Cattanach L, Rodin J: Psychosocial components of the stress process in bulimia. Int J Eating Disord 1988; 7:75-88

57. Chatfield WR, Bowditch JDP, Forrest CA: Spontaneous pneumomediastinum complicating anorexia nervosa. Br Med J 1979; 1:200-201

58. Chattem Professional Services: Pamabrom and pyrilamine maleate. Two of the active ingredients in Premesyn PMS™. Booklet. Chatanooga, TN, Chattem, Inc, 1985

59. Chiodo J: The assessment of anorexia nervosa and bulimia. Prog Behav Modif 1985; 19:255-92

60. Chiodo J, Latimer PR: Hunger perceptions and satiety responses among normal-weight bulimics and normals to a high-calorie, carbohydrate-rich food. Psychol Med 1986; 16:343-349

61. Chiodo J, Latimer PR: Vomiting as a learned weight-control technique in bulimia. J Behav Ther Exp Psychiat 1983; 14:131-135

62. Clark DC: Oral complications of anorexia nervosa and/or bulimia: With a review of the literature. J Oral Med 1985; 40:134-138

63. Clark JE, Simon WA: Cardiac arrhythmias after phenylpropanolamine ingestion. Drug Intell Clin Pharm 1983; 17:737-738

64. Clarke MG, Palmer RL: Eating attitudes and neurotic symptoms in university students. Br J Psychiatry 1983; 142:299-304

65. Collins JK, Beumont JJV, Touyz SW, et al: Variability in body shape perception in anorexic, bulimic, obese, and control subjects. Int J Eating Disord 1987; 6:633-638

66. Connors ME, Johnson CL, Stuckey MK: Treatment of bulimia with brief psychoeducation group therapy. Am J Psychiatry 1984; 141:1512-1516

67. Cooke WT: Laxative abuse. Clin Gastroenterol 1977; 6:659-673

68. Cooper PJ, Charnock DJ, Taylor MJ: The prevalence of bulimia nervosa: A replication study. Br J Psychiatry 1987; 151:684-686

69. Cooper PJ, Fairburn CG: Binge-eating and self-induced vomiting in the community – A preliminary study. Br J Psychiatry 1983; 142:139–144

70. Cooper PJ, Fairburn CG: The depressive symptoms of bulimia nervosa. Br J Psychiatry 1986; 148:268–274

71. Cooper JL, Morrison TL, Bigman OL, et al: Bulimia and borderline personality disorder. Int J Eating Disord 1988; 7:43–49

72. Cooper JL, Morrison TL, Bigman OL, et al: Mood changes and affective disorder in the binge-purge cycle. Int J Eating Disord 1988; 7:469–474

73. Cooper PJ, Waterman GC, Fairburn CG: Women with eating problems: A community survey. Br J Clin Psychol 1984; 23:45–52

74. Coovert DL, Powers PS: Bulimia nervosa with enema abuse: A preliminary analysis based on four case reports. Int J Eating Disord 1988; 7:697–700

75. Copeland PM, Herzog DB: Non-Bulimia: Food regurgitation in a patient with self-diagnosed bulimia. J Clin Psychiatry 1986; 47:317–318

76. Cuellar RE, Van Thiel DH: Gastrointestinal consequences of eating disorders: Anorexia nervosa and bulimia. Am J Gastroenterol 1986; 81:1113–1124

77. Cuellar RE, Tarter R, Hays A, et al: The possible occurrence of "alcoholic hepatitis" in a patient with bulimia in the absence of diagnosable alcoholism. Hepatology 1987; 7:878–883

78. Cummings JH: Progress report: Laxative abuse. Gut 1974; 15:758–766

79. Cuthbert MF: Anorectic and decongestant preparations containing phenylpropanolamine. Lancet 1980; 1:60

80. Davidson C, Silverstone T: Diuretic dependence. Br Med J 1972; 282:505

81. de Wardener HE: Idiopathic edema: Role of diuretic abuse. Kidney Int 1981; 19:881–92

82. Diagnostic and Statistical Manual of Mental Disorders (third edition revised), APA, 1985

83. Dickstein LJ: Anorexia nervosa and bulimia: A review of clinical issues. Hosp Community Psychiatry 1985; 36:1086–1091

84. Dietz AJ: Amphetamine-like reactions to phenylpropanolamine. JAMA 1981; 245:601–602

85. Donley AJ, Kemple TJ: Spontaneous pneumomediastinum complicating anorexia nervosa. Br Med J 1978; 11:1604–1605

86. Drewnowski A, Halmi KA, Pierce B, et al: Taste and eating disorders. Am J Clin Nutr 1987; 46:442–450

87. Drewnowski A, Pierce B, Halmi KA: Fat aversion in eating disorders. Appetite 1988; 10:119–131

88. Drewnowski A, Hopkins SA, Kessler RC: The prevalence of bulimia nervosa in the US college student population. Am J Public Health 1988; 78:1322–1325

89. Eckert ED, Goldberg SC, Halmi KA, et al: Depression in anorexia nervosa. Psychol Med 1982; 12:115–122

90. Eckert ED, Halmi KA, Marchi P, et al: Comparison of bulimic and non-bulimic anorexia nervosa patients during treatment. Psychol Med 1987; 17:891–898

91. Edelstein C, Roy-Byrne P, Fawzy FI, et al: Effects of weight loss on the dexamethasone suppression test. American Psychiatric Association Annual Meeting Abstract, New York, 1983

92. Edwards FE, Nagelberg DB: Personality characteristics of restrained/binge eaters versus unrestrained/nonbinge eaters. Addict Behav 1986; 11:207–211

93. Edwards GM: Case of bulimia nervosa presenting with acute, fatal abdominal distension. Lancet 1985; 1:822–823

94. Edwards OM, Bayliss RIS: Idiopathic oedema of women. J Med 1976; 45:125–144

95. Fairburn C: A cognitive behavioural approach to the treatment of bulimia. Psychol Med 1981; 11:707–711

96. Fairburn CG: Binge-eating and bulmia nervosa. SK&F Publications, vol 1, 1982, pp 1–20

97. Fairburn CG: Binge-eating and its management. Br J Psychiatry 1982; 141:631–633

98. Fairburn CG: Bulimia: Its epidemiology and management. In Eating and Its Disorders. Edited by Stunkard AJ, Steller E. New York: Raven, 1983

99. Fairburn CG: The definition of bulimia nervosa: Guidelines for clinicians and research workers. Ann Behavior Med 1987; 9:3–7

100. Fairburn CG: Self-induced vomiting. J Psychosom Res 1980; 24:193–197

101. Fairburn CG: The management of bulimia nervosa. J Psychiatr Res 1985; 19:465–472

102. Fairburn CG, Cooper PJ: Binge-eating, self-induced vomiting and laxative abuse: A community study. Psychol Med 1984; 14:401–410

103. Fairburn CG, Cooper PJ: Self-induced vomiting and bulimia nervosa: An undetected problem. Br Med J 1982; 284:1153–1155

104. Fairburn CG, Cooper PJ, Kirk J, et al: The significance of the neurotic symptoms of bulimia nervosa. J Psychiatr Res 1985; 19:135–140

105. Fairburn CG, Garner DM: The diagnosis of bulimia nervosa. Int J Eating Disord 1986; 1–28

106. Fairburn CG, Kirk J, O'Connor M, et al: A comparison of two psychological treatments for bulimia nervosa. Behav Res Ther, (in press)

107. Fairburn CG, Kirk J, O'Connor M, et al: Prognostic factors in bulimia nervosa. Br J Clin Psychology 1987; 26:223–224

108. Ferguson JM: Bulimia: A potentially fatal syndrome. Psychosomatics 1985; 26:252–253

109. Ferguson JM: Habits not diets: The real way to weight control. Palo Alto, California: Bull Publishing, 1976

110. Fichter MM, Pirke KM, Pollinger J, et al: Restricted caloric intake causes neuroendocrine disturbances in bulimia, in The Psychobiology of Bulimia. Edited by Pirke KM, Vandereycken W, Ploog D. Berlin: Springer-Verlag, 1988

111. Finton CK, Barton M, Chernow B: Possible adverse effects of phenylpropanolamine (diet pills) on sympathetic nervous system function-caveat emptor. Milit Med 1982; 147:1072

112. Food and Drug Administration: Orally administered menstrual drug products for over-the-counter human use: Monograph. Fed Register 1982; 47:199

113. Freeman CPL, Barry F, Dunkeld-Turnbull J, et al: Controlled trial of psychotherapy for bulimia nervosa. Br Med J 1988; 296:521–525

114. Freeman CPL, Hampson M: Fluoxetine as a treatment for bulimia nervosa. Int J Obes 1987; 11:171–177

115. Friedman EJ: Death from ipecac intoxication in a patient with anorexia-nervosa. Am J Psychiatry 1984; 141:702–703

116. Frier BM: Osteomalacia and arthropathy associated with prolonged abuse of purgatives. Br J Clin Prac 1977; 31:17–19

117. Fullerton DT, Swift WJ, Getto CJ, et al: Differences in the plasma beta-endorphin levels of bulimics. Int J Eating Disord 1988; 7:191–200

118. Fullerton DT, Swift WJ, Getto CJ, et al: Plasma immunoreactive beta-endorphin in bulimics. Psychol Med 1986; 16:59–63

119. Garfinkel PE, Garner DM: Anorexia nervosa: A multidimensional perspective. New York: Brunner/Mazel, 1982

120. Garfinkel PE, Moldofsky H, Gardner DM: The heterogeneity of anorexia nervosa: Bulimia as a distinct subgroup. Arch Gen Psychiatry 1980; 37:1036–1040

121. Garner DM: Individual psychotherapy for anorexia nervosa. J Psychiatr Res 1985; 19:423–433

122. Garner DM, Fairburn CG, Davis R: Cognitive-Behavioral treatment of bulimia nervosa: A critical appraisal. Behav Mod 1987; 4:398–431

123. Garner DM, Garfinkel PE, O'Shaughnessy M: The validity of the distinction between bulimia with and without anorexia nervosa. Am J Psychiatry 1985; 142:581–587

124. Garner DM, Garfinkel PE, O'Shaughness M: Clinical and psychometric comparison be-

tween bulimia in anorexia and bulimia in normal-weight women. Report of the Fourth Ross Conference on Medical Research 1983; 6–11

125. Garner DM, Garfinkel PE, Schwartz D, et al: Cultural expectations of thinness in women. Psychol Rep 1980; 47:483–491.

126. Garner DM, Olmsted MP, Garfinkel PE: Similarities among bulimic groups selected by different weights and weight histories. J Psychiatr Res 1985; 19:129–134

127. Gavish D, Eisenberg S, Berry EM, et al: An underlying behavioral disorder in hyperlipidemic pancreatitis: A prospective multidisciplinary approach. Arch Intern Med 1987; 147:705–708

128. Geracioti TD, Liddle RA: Impaired cholecystokinin secretion in bulimia nervosa. N Engl J Med 1988; 319:683–688

129. Gerlinghoff M, Backmund H: Kleptomanie bei anorexia nervosa und bulimie. Mschr Krim 1986; 69:325–331

130. Gerlinghoff M, Backmund H: Stehlen bei anorexia nervosa and bulimia nervosa. Fortschr Neurol Psychiatr 1987; 55:343–346

131. Gerner RH, Gwirtsman HE: Abnormalities of dexamethasone suppression test and urinary MHPG in anorexia nervosa. Am J Psychiatry 1981; 138:650–653

132. Gilinsky NH, Humphries LL, Fried AM, et al: Computed tomographic abnormalities of the pancreas in eating disorders: A report of two cases with normal laparotomy. Int J Eating Disord 1988; 7:567–572

133. Goldberg SG, Eckert ED, Halmi KA, et al: Effects of cyproheptadine on symptoms and attitudes in anorexia nervosa. Arch Gen Psychiatry 1980; 30:1083

134. Goode ET: Medical aspects of the bulimic syndrome and bulimarexia. Transact Analysis J 1985; 15:4–11

135. Grace PS, Jacobson RS, Fullager CJ: A pilot comparison of purging and non-purging bulimics. J Clin Psychol 1985; 41:173–180

136. Gray JJ, Ford K: The incidence of bulimia in a college sample. Int J Eating Disord 1985; 2:201–210

137. Green RS, Rau JH: Treatment of compulsive eating disturbances with anticonvulsant medication. Am J Psychiatry 1974; 131:428–432

138. Greenway FL, Bray GA: Cholecystokinin and satiety. Life Sci 1977; 21:769–771

139. Griboff SI, Berman R, Siverman HI: A double-blind clinical evaluation of a phenylpropanolamine-caffeine-vitamin combination and a placebo in the treatment of exogenous obesity. Curr Ther Res 1975; 17:535–543

140. Gross DJ, Chetrit EB, Stein P, et al: Edema associated with laxative abuse and excessive diuretic therapy. Isr J Med Sci 1980; 16:787–789

141. Gross HA, Lake CR, Ebert MH, et al: Catecholamine metabolism in primary anorexia nervosa. J Clin Endocrinol Metab 1979; 49:805–809

142. Gross M: Aspects of bulimia. Cleve Clin Q 1983; 50:19–25

143. Guiora AZ: Dysorexia: A psychopathological study of anorexia nervosa and bulimia. Am J Psychiatry 1967; 124:391–393

144. Gupta MA, Gupta AK, Haberman HF: Dermatologic signs in anorexia nervosa and bulimia nervosa. Arch Dermatol 1987; 123:1386–1390

145. Gwirtsman HE, Roy-Byrne P, Yager J, et al: Neuroendocrine abnormalities in bulimia. Am J Psychiatry 1983; 140:559–563

146. Gwirtsman HE, Yager J, Gillard BK, et al: Serum amylase and its isoenzymes in normal weight bulimia. Int J Eating Disord 1986; 5:355–361

147. Halmi KA: Catecholamine metabolism in anorexia nervosa. Int J Psychiatry Med 1981; 11:251–254

148. Halmi KA: Classification of eating disorders. Int J Eating Disord 1983; 2:21–26

149. Halmi KA, Dekirmenjian H, Davis JM, et al: Catecholamine metabolism in anorexia nervosa. Arch Gen Psychiatry 1978; 35:458–460

150. Halmi KA, Eckert E, Falk JR: Cyproheptadine, an antidepressant and weight inducing drug for anorexia nervosa. Psychopharmacol Bull 1983; 19:103–105

151. Halmi KA, Eckert E, LaDu TJ, et al: Treatment efficacy of cyproheptadine and amitriptyline. Arch Gen Psychiatry 1986; 43:177–181

152. Halmi KA, Falk JR, Schwartz E: Binge eating and vomiting: A survey of a college population. Pyschol Med 1981; 11:697–706

153. Hart KJ, Ollendick TH: Prevalence of bulimia in working and university women. Am J Psychiatry 1985; 142:851–854

154. Hatsukami D, Owen P, Pyle R, et al: Similarities and differences on the MMPI between women with bulimia and women with alcohol or drug abuse problems. Addict Behav 1982; 7:435–439

155. Hatsukami D, Eckert E, Mitchell JE, et al: Affective disorders and substance abuse in women with bulimia. Psychol Med 1984; 14:701–704

156. Hatsukami DK, Mitchell JE, Eckert ED: Eating disorders: A variant of mood disorder? Psychiatr Clin North Am 1984; 7:349–365

157. Hatsukami D, Mitchell JE, Eckert ED, et al: Characteristics of patients with bulimia only, bulimia with affective disorder, and bulimia with substance abuse problems. Addict Behav 1986; 11:399–406

158. Hawkins II, Clement PF: Development and construct validation of a self-reported measure of binge eating tendencies. Addict Behav 1980; 5:219–226

159. Hendren RL, Barber JK, Sigafoos A: Eating-disordered symptoms in a nonclinical population: A study of female adolescents in two private schools. J Am Acad Child Psychiatry 1986; 25:836–840

160. Herman CP, Polivy J: Restraint and excess in dieters and bulimics, in The Psychobiology of Bulimia. Edited by Pirke KM, Vandereycken W, Ploog D. Berlin: Springer-Verlag, 1988

161. Herzog DB: Are anorexic and bulimic patients depressed? Am J Psychiatry 1984; 141:1594–1597

162. Herzog DB: Bulimia in the adolescent. Am J Dis Child 1982; 136:985–989

163. Herzog DB: Bulimia: The secretive syndrome. Psychosomatics 1982; 23:481–487

164. Herzog DB, Norman DK, Gordon C, et al: Sexual conflict and eating disorders in 27 males. Am J Psychiatry 1984; 141:989–990

165. Herzog DB, Norman DK, Rigotti NA, et al: Frequency of bulimic behaviors and associated social maladjustment in female graduate students. J Psychiatr Res 1986; 20:355–361

166. Herzog DB, Keller MB, Lavori PW: Outcome in anorexia nervosa and bulimia nervosa: A review of the literature. J Nerv Ment Dis 1988; 176:131–143

167. Herzog DB, Keller MB, Lavori PW: Social impairment in bulimia. Int J Eating Disord 1987; 6:741–747

168. Herzog DB, Keller MB, Lavori PW, et al: Short-term prospective study of recovery in bulimia nervosa. Psychiatry Res 1988; 23:45–55

169. Herzog DB, Pepose M, Norman DK, et al: Eating disorders and social maladjustment in female medical students. J Nerv Ment Dis 1985; 173:734–737

170. Hillard JR, Lobo MC, Keeling RP: Bulimia and diabetes: A potentially life-threatening combination. Psychosomatics 1983; 24:292–295

171. Hinz LD, Williamson DA: Bulimia and Depression: A review of the affective variant hypothesis. Psychol Bull 1987; 102:150–158

172. Hoffman JJ: A double blind crossover clinical trial of an OTC diuretic in the treatment of premenstrual tension and weight gain. Curr Ther Res 1979; 26:575–580

173. Hohlstein LA, Gwirtsman HE, Whalen F, et al: Oral glucose tolerance in bulimia. Int J Eating Disord 1986; 5:157-160

174. Hollister LE, Johnson K, Bookhabza D, et al: Adverse effects of naltrexone in subjects not dependent on opiates. Drug Alcohol Depend 1981; 8:37-41

175. Holtzman SG: Behavioral effects of separate and combined administration of naloxone and d-amphetamine. J Pharm Exp Ther 1974; 189:51-60

176. Horne RL, Ferguson JM, Pope HG, et al: Treatment of bulimia with bupropion: A multicenter controlled trial. J Clin Psychiatry 1988; 49:262-266

177. House RC, Bliziotes MM, Licht JH: Perimolysis: Unveiling the surreptitious vomiter. Oral Surg 1981; 51:152-155

178. Hsu LK: Treatment of bulimia with lithium. Am J Psychiatry 1984; 141:1260-1262

179. Hsu LKG, Holder D: Bulimia nervosa: Treatment and short-term outcome. Psychol Med 1986; 16:65-70

180. Hudson JI, Hudson MS: Endocrine dysfunction in anorexia nervosa and bulimia: Comparison with abnormalities in other psychiatric disorders and disturbances due to metabolic factors. Psychiatr Devel 1984; 4:237-272

181. Hudson JI, Hudson MS, Wentworth SM: Self-induced glycosuria: A novel method of purging in bulimia. JAMA 1983; 249:2501

182. Hudson JI, Katz DL, Pope HG, et al: Urinary free cortisol and response to the dexamethasone suppression test in bulima: A pilot study. Int J Eating Disord 1987; 6:191-198

183. Hudson JI, Laffer PS, Pope HG: Bulimia related to affective disorder by family history and response to the dexamethasone suppression test. Am J Psychiatry 1982; 139:685-687

184. Hudson JI, Pope HG Jr: Depression and eating disorders. In OG Cameron (Ed), Presentations of depression: Symptoms of depression in medical and other psychiatric disorders 1987; pp. 33-66, New York: Wiley

185. Hudson JI, Pope HG Jr: Newer antidepressants in the treatment of bulimia. Psychopharmacol Bull 1987; 23:52-57

186. Hudson JI, Pope HG, Jonas JM: Psychosis in anorexia nervosa and bulimia. Br J Psychiatry 1984; 145:420-423

187. Hudson JI, Pope HG, Jonas JM, et al: A controlled family history study of bulimia. Psychol Med 1987; 17:883-890

188. Hudson JI, Pope, HG Jr, Jonas JM, et al: Family history study of anorexia nervosa and bulimia. Br J Psychiatry 1983; 142:133-138

189. Hudson JI, Pope HG, Jonas JM, et al: Phenomenologic relationship of eating disorders to major affective disorder. Psychiatry Res 1983; 9:345-54

190. Hudson JI, Pope HG, Jonas JM, et al: Sleep EEG in bulimia. Biol Psychiatry 1987; 22:820-828

191. Hudson JI, Pope HG, Wurtman J, et al: Bulimia in obese individuals: Relationship to normal-weight bulimia. J Nerv Ment Dis 1988; 176:144-152

192. Hudson JI, Pope HG, Yurgelun-Todd, D, et al: A controlled study of lifetime prevalence of affective and other psychiatric disorders in bulimic outpatients. Am J Psychiatry 1987; 144:1283-1287

193. Hudson JI, Weiss RD, Pope HG, et al: Eating disorders in hospitalized substance abusers. J Clin Psychiatry (in press).

194. Hudson MS, Wentworth SM: Bulimia and diabetes. N Engl J Med 1983; 309:431-432

195. Hudson JI, Wentworth SM, Hudson MS, et al: Prevalence of anorexia nervosa and bulimia among young diabetic women. J Clin Psychiatry 1985; 46:88-89

196. Hughes PL, Wells LA, Cunningham CJ, et al: Treating bulimia with desipramine. Arch Gen Psychiatry 1986; 43:182-186

197. Hughes PL, Wells LA, Cunningham CJ: The dexamethasone suppression test in bulimia before and after successful treatment with desipramine. J Clin Psychiatry 1986; 47:515–517

198. Humphries L, Shih WJ: Gastric emptying time in anorexia nervosa and bulimia. Arch Surg 1988; 123:783

199. Huon GF, Brown LB: Body images in anorexia nervosa and bulimia nervosa. Int J Eating Disord 1986; 5:421–439

200. Hurst PS, Lacey JH, Crisp AH: Teeth, vomiting and diet: A study of the dental characteristics of seventeen anorexia nervosa patients. Postgrad Med 1977; 53:298–305

201. Igoin-Apfelbaum L, Apfelbaum M: Naltrexone and bulimic symptoms. Lancet 1987; 1–87–1088

202. Isner JM: Effects of ipecac on the heart. N Engl J Med 1986; 314:1253

203. Jacobs MB, Schneider JA: Medical complications of bulimia: A prospective evaluation. Q J Med 1985; 54:177–182

204. James EC: Postemetic rupture of herniated cardia of the stomach. JAMA 1984; 251:471

205. Jamison RL, Ross JC, Kempson RL, et al: Surreptitious diuretic ingestion and pseudo-Bartter's syndrome. Am J Med 1982; 73:142–147

206. Jimerson DC, Brandt HA, Brewerton TD: Evidence for altered serotonin function in bulimia and anorexia nervosa: Behavioral implications, in The Psychobiology of Bulimia. Edited by Pirke KM, Vandereycken W, Ploog D. Berlin: Springer-Verlag, 1988

207. Jimerson DC, George DT, Kaye WH, et al: Norepinephrine regulation in bulimia. In The Psychobiology of Bulimia. Edited by Hudson JI, Pope HG. Washington, DC: American Psychiatric Press, Inc., 1987

208. Jirik-Babb P, Katz JL: Impairment of taste perception in anorexia nervosa and bulimia. Int J Eating Disord 1988; 7:353–360

209. Johnson C, Berndt DJ: Preliminary investigations of bulimia and life adjustment. Am J Psychiatry 140:774–777, 1983

210. Johnson C, Connors M, Stuckey M: Short-term group treatment of bulimia: A preliminary report. Int J Eating Disord 1983; 2:199–208

211. Johnson C, Flach A: Family characteristics of 105 patients with bulimia. Am J Psychiatry 1985; 142:1321–1324

212. Johnson C, Larson R: Bulimia: an analysis of moods and behavior. Psychosom Med 44:341–351, 1982

213. Johnson C, Maddi KL: The etiology of bulimia: A bio-psycho-social perspective. Adolesc Psychiatry 1986; 13:253–73

214. Johnson C, Tobin D, Enright A: Prevalence and clinical characteristics of borderline patients in an eating disordered population. J Clin Psychiatry (in press)

215. Johnson CL, Lewis G, Love S, et al: A descriptive survey of dieting and bulimic behavior in a female high school population, in Understanding Anorexia Nervosa and Bulimia. Columbus, Ohio: Ross Laboratories, 1983, pp 14–18

216. Johnson CL, Stuckey MK, Lewis LD, et al: Bulimia: A descriptive survey of 316 cases. Int J Eating Disord 1982; 2:3–16

217. Johnson DA, Eitter HS, Reeves D: Stroke and phenylpropanolamine use. Lancet 1983; 2:970

218. Johnson DL, Rue VM: The bulimic dental patient: Recognition and recommendations. Dent Hygiene 1985; 59:372–377

219. Johnson GL, Humphries LL, Shirley PB, et al: Mitral valve prolapse in patients with anorexia nervosa and bulimia. Arch Intern Med 1986; 146:1525–1529

220. Jonas D, Gold MS: Naltrexone reverses bulimic symptoms. Lancet 1986; 1:807

221. Jonas JM, Gold MS: Opiate antagonists as clinical probes in bulimia. The Psychobiology of Bulimia. Edited by Hudson JI, Pope HG. Washington, DC: American Psychiatric Press, Inc., 1987

222. Jonas JM, Gold MS, Sweeney D, et al: Eating disorders and cocaine abuse: A survey of 259 cocaine abusers. J Clin Psychiatry 1987; 48:47–50

223. Jones DA, Cheshire N, Moorhouse H: Anorexia nervosa, bulimia and alcoholism—Association of eating disorder and alcohol. J Psychiat Res 1985; 19:377–380

224. Joseph AB, Herr B: Finger calluses in bulimia. Am J Psychiatry 1985; 142:655

225. Kagan DM, Squires RL: Eating disorders among adolescents: Patterns and prevalence. Adolescence 1984; 19:15–29

226. Kaminer Y, Feingold M, Lyons K: Single Case Study: Bulimia in a pair of monozygotic twins. J Nerv Ment Dis 1988; 176:246–248

227. Kaplan AS: Hyperamylasemia and bulimia: A clinical review. Int J Eating Disord 1987; 6:537–543

228. Kaplan AS: Thyroid function in bulimia. In The Psychobiology of Bulimia, JI Hudson and HG Pope (Eds). Washington, DC: American Psychiatric Press, 1987

229. Kaplan AS, Garfinkel PE, Warsh JJ, et al: The DST and TRH stimulation test in normal weight bulimia. Presented at the 2nd International Conference on Eating Disorders, New York, April 1986

230. Kaplan AS, Garfinkel PE, Garner DM: Bulimia treated with carbamazepine and imipramine. Presented at the American Psychiatric Association Meeting, Chicago, 1987

231. Katzman MA, Wolchik SA: Bulimia and binge-eating in college women: A comparison of personality and behavioral characteristics. J Consult Clin Psychol 1984; 52:423–428

232. Katzman MA, Wolchik SA, Braver SL: The prevalence of frequent binge eating and bulimia in a nonclinical college sample. Int J Eating Disord 1984; 3:53–62

233. Kaye WH, Ebert MH, Gwirtsman, HE, et al: Differences in brain serotonergic metabolism between nonbulimic and bulimic patients with anorexia nervosa. Am J Psychiatry 1984; 141:1598–1601

234. Kaye WH, Gwirtsman HE, Brewerton TD, et al: Bingeing behavior and plasma amino acids: A possible involvement of brain serotonin in bulimia nervosa. Psychiatr Res 1988; 23:31–43

235. Kaye WH, Rubinow D, Gwirtsman HE, et al: CSF somatostatin in anorexia nervosa and bulimia: Relationship to the hypothalamic pituitary-adrenal cortical axis. Psychoneuroendocrinology 1988; 13:1–8

236. Keefe PH, Wyshogrod D, Weinberger E, et al: Binge-eating and outcome of behavioral treatment of obesity: A preliminary report. Behav Res Ther 1984; 22:319–321

237. Kelly JT, Patten SE, Johannes A: Analysis of self-reported eating and related behaviors in an adolescent population. Nutr Res 1982; 2:417–432

238. Kerr WF: Spontaneous intramural rupture and intramural hematoma of the oesophagus. Thorax 1980; 35:890–897

239. Keys A, Brozek J, Henschel AJ, et al: The Biology of Human Starvation. Minneapolis, University of Minnesota Press, 1950

240. Kikta DG, Devereaux MW, Chandar K: Intracranial hemorrhages due to phenylpropanolamine. Stroke 1985; 16:510–512

241. Killen JD, Taylor CB, Telch MJ, et al: Depressive symptoms and substance use among adolescent binge eaters and purgers: A defined population study. Am J Public Health 1987; 77:1539–1541

242. Killen JD, Taylor B, Telch MJ, et al: Self-induced vomiting and laxative and diuretic use among teenagers. Precursors of the binge-purge syndrome? JAMA 1986; 255:1447–1449

243. Kim SK, Gerle RD, Rozanski R: Cathartic colitis. Am J Roentgenology 1978; 131:1079–1081

244. Kiriike N, Nishiwaki S, Izumiya Y, et al: Dexamethasone suppression test in bulimia. Biol Psychiatry 1986; 21:325–328

245. Kirkley BG, Schneider JA, Agras WS, et al: Comparison of two group treatments for bulimia. J Consult Clin Psychology 1985; 53:43–48

246. Kissileff HR, Walsh BT, Kral JG, et al: Laboratory studies of eating behavior in women with bulimia. Physiol Behav 1986; 38:563–570

247. Kiyohara K, Tamai H, Karibe C, et al: Serum thyrotropin (TSH) responses to thyrotropin-releasing hormone (TRH) in patients with anorexia nervosa and bulimia: Influence of changes in body weight and eating disorders. Psychoneuroendocrinology 1987; 12:21–28

248. Kog E, Vandereycken W, Vertommen H: Towards a verification of the psychosomatic family model: A pilot study of ten families with anorexia/bulimia nervosa patient. Int J Eating Disord 1985; 4:525–538

249. Kog E, Vandereycken W: Family characteristics of anorexia nervosa and bulimia: A review of the research literature. Clin Psychol Rev 1985; 5:159–180

250. Krahn D, Mitchell JE: Tryptophan ineffective in bulimia. Am J Psychiatry 1985; 142:1130

251. Krieg JC: Cranial computed tomography findings in patients with eating disorder, in The Psychobiology of Bulimia. Edited by Pirke KM, Vandereycken W, Ploog D. Berlin: Springer-Verlag, 1988

252. Lacey JH: Bulimia nervosa, binge eating, and psychogenic vomiting: A controlled treatment study and long term outcome. Br Med J 1983; 286:1609–1613

253. Lacey JH, Coker S, Birtchnell SA: Bulimia: Factors associated with its etiology and maintenance. Int J Eating Disord 1986; 5:475–487

254. Lacey JH, Gibson E: Controlling weight by purgation and vomiting: A comparative study of bulimics. J Psychiatr Res 1985; 19:337–341

255. Lacey JH, Gibson E: Does laxative abuse control body weight? A comparative study of purging and vomiting bulimics. Hum Nutr Appl Nutr 1985; 39A:36–42

256. Lacey JH, Moureli E: Bulimic alcoholics: Some features of a clinical sub-group. Br J Addict 1986; 81:389–393

257. Laessle RG, Kittl S, Fichter MM, et al: Major affective disorder in anorexia nervosa and bulimia: A descriptive diagnostic study. Br J Psychyiatry 1987; 151:785–789

258. Lankenau H, Swigar ME, Bhimani S, et al: Cranial CT scans in eating disorder patients and controls. Compr Psychiatry 1985; 26:136–147

259. Larocca FE, Della-Fera MA: Rumination: Its significance in adults with bulimia nervosa. Psychosomatics 1986; 27:209–212

260. Larsen K, Jensen BS, Axelsen F: Perforation and rupture of the esophagus. Scand J Thorac Cardiovasc Surg 1983; 17:311–316

261. Larusso NF, McGill DB: Surreptitious laxative ingestion: Delayed recognition of a serious condition: A case report. Mayo Clin Proc 1975; 50:706–708

262. Lasagna L: Phenylpropanolamine and blood pressure. JAMA 1985; 253:2491–2492

263. Lee KY, Vandogen R, Beilin LJ: Severe hypertension after ingestion of an appetite suppressant (phenylpropanolamine) with indomethacin. Lancet 1979; 1:1110–1111

264. Lee NL, Rush AJ: Cognitive-behavioral group therapy for bulimia. Int J Eating Disord 1986; 5:599–615

265. Lee NL, Ruch AJ, Mitchell JE: Depression and bulimia. J Affect Disord 1985; 9:231–238

266. Leibowitz SF: Brain monoamines and peptides: Role in the control of eating behavior. Fed Pro 1986; 45:1396–1403

267. Leitenberg H, Gross J, Peterson J, et al: Analysis of an anxiety model and the process of change during exposure plus response prevention treatment of bulimia nervosa. Behav Ther 15:13–20, 1984

268. Leitenberg H, Rosen JC, Gross J, et al: Exposure plus response-prevention treatment of bulimia nervosa. J Consult Clin Psychol 1988; 56:535–541

269. Leon GR, Carroll K, Chernyk B, et al: Binge-eating and associated habit patterns within college student and identified bulimic populations. Int J Eating Disord 1985; 4:43–57

270. Lesna M, Hamlyn AN, Venables CW, et al: Chronic laxative abuse associated with pancreatic islet cell hyperplasia. Gut 1977; 18:1032–1035

271. Levin AP, Hyler SE: DSM-III personality diagnosis in bulimia. Compr Psychiatry 1986; 27:47–53

272. Levin PA, Falko JM, Dixon K, et al: Benign parotid enlargement in bulimia. Ann Intern Med 1980; 93:827–829

273. Levine DF, Wingat DL, Pfeffer J, et al: Habitual rumination: a benign disorder. Br Med J 1983; 287:255–256

274. Levy AB, Dixon KN: DST in bulimia without endogenous depression. Biol Psychiatry 1987; 22:783–786

275. Levy AB, Dixon KN, Schmidt H: Sleep architecture in anorexia nervosa and bulimia. Biol Psychiatry 1988; 23:99–101

276. Lindy DC, Walsh BT, Roose SP, et al: The dexamethasone suppression test in bulimia. Am J Psychiatry 1985; 142:1375–1376

277. Lombrose CT, Schwartz IH, Clark DM: Ctenoids in healthy youths. Neurology 1966; 16:1152–1158

278. Long MT, Johnson LC: Fourteen- and six-per-second positive spikes in a nonclinical male population. Neurology 1968; 18:714–716

279. Lowy MT, Maickel RP, Yim GKW: Naloxone reduction of stress-related feeding. Life Sci 1980; 26:2113–2118

280. Lundholm JK, Anderson DF: Eating disordered behaviors: A comparison of male and female university students. Addict Behav 1986; 11:193–196

281. MacGregor GA, Markandu ND, Roulston JE, et al: Is "idiopathic" oedema idiopathic? Lancet 1979; 1:397–400

282. MacGregor GA, Tasker PRW, de Wardener HE: Diuretic induced oedema. Lancet 1975; I:489–492

283. Maggio CA, Presta E, Bracco EF: Naltrexone and human eating behavior: A dose-ranging inpatient trial in moderately obese men. Brain Res Bull 1985; 14:657–661

284. Malcom R, O'Neil PM, Sexauer JD: A controlled trial of naltrexone in obese humans. Int J Obes 1985; 9:347–353

285. Manno BR, Manno JE: Toxicology of ipecac: A review. Clinical Toxicol 1977; 10, 221–242

286. Marcus MD, Wing RR, Lamparski DM: Binge-eating and dietary restraint in obese patients. Addict Behav 1985; 10:163–168

287. Martin WR, Wickler A, Edes CG, et al: Tolerance to and physical dependence on morphine in rats. Psychopharmacol 1963; 4:247–260

288. Maulsby RL: EEG patterns of uncertain diagnostic significance, in Current Practice of Clinical Electroencephalography. Edited by Klass DW, Daly DD. New York: Raven Press, 1979; pp 411–419

289. Meermann R, Vandereycken W: Body image disturbances in eating disorders from the viewpoint of experimental research, in The Psychobiology of Bulimia Nervosa. Edited by Pirke KM, Vandereycken W, Ploog D. Germany: Springer-Verlag, 1988; pp 158–171

290. Michel L: Post-emetic laceration and rupture of the gastroesophageal junction. Acta Chir Belg 1982; 1:13–24

291. Mitchell JE: Bulimia with self-induced vomiting after gastric stapling. Am J Psychiatry 1985; 142:656

292. Mitchell JE: Medical complications of anorexia nervosa and bulimia. Psychiatr Med 1983; 1:229–256

293. Mitchell JE, Bantle JP: Metabolic and endocrine investigations in women of normal weight with the bulimia syndrome. Biol Psychiatry 1983; 18:355–365

294. Mitchell JE, Boutacoff LI: Laxative abuse complicating bulimia: Medical and treatment implications. Int J Eating Disord 1986; 5:325–334

295. Mitchell JE, Boutacoff LI, Hatsukami D, et al: Laxative abuse as a variant of bulimia. J Nerv Ment Dis 1986; 174:174–176

296. Mitchell JE, Davis L, Goff G: The process of relapse in patients with bulimia. Int J Eating Disord 1985; 4:457–463

297. Mitchell JE, Davis, L, Goff G, et al: A follow-up study of patients with bulimia. Int J Eating Disord 1986; 5:441–450

298. Mitchell JE, Goff G: Bulimia in male patients. Psychosomatics 1984; 25:909–913

299. Mitchell JE, Groat R: A placebo-controlled, double-blind trial of amitriptyline in bulimia. J Clin Psychopharmacol 1984; 4:186–193

300. Mitchell JE, Hatsukami D, Eckert ED, et al: Characteristics of 275 patients with bulimia. Am J Psychiatry 1985; 142:482–485

301. Mitchell JE, Hatsukami D, Eckert E, et al: Eating Disorders Questionnaire. Psychopharmacol Bull 1985; 21:1025–1043

302. Mitchell JE, Hatsukami D, Pyle RL, et al: Late onset bulimia. Compr Psychiatry 1987; 28:323–328

303. Mitchell JE, Hatsukami D, Pyle RL, et al: The bulimia syndrome: Course of the illness and associated problems. Compr Psychiatry 1986; 27:165–170

304. Mitchell JE, Hosfield W, Pyle RL: EEG findings in patients with the bulimia syndrome. Int J Eating Disord 1983; 2:17–23

305. Mitchell JE, Laine DC: Monitored binge-eating behavior in patients with bulimia. Int J Eating Disord 1985; 4:177–183

306. Mitchell JE, Laine DC, Morley JE, et al: Naloxone but not CCK-8 may attenuate binge-eating behavior in patients with bulimia syndrome. Biol Psychiatry 1986; 21:1399–1406

307. Mitchell JE, Morley JE: Endogenous opioid peptides and feeding, in The Psychobiology of Bulimia. Edited by Hudson JI, Pope HG. Washington, DC: American Psychiatric Press, Inc., 1987; pp 101–113

308. Mitchell JE, Morley JE, Levine AS, et al: High-dose naltrexone therapy and dietary counseling for obesity. Biol Psychiatry 1987; 22:35–42

309. Mitchell JE, Pomery C, Huber M: A clinician's guide to the eating disorders medicine cabinet. Int J Eating Disord 1988; 2:211–223

310. Mitchell JE, Pomeroy C, Seppala M, et al: Diuretic use as a marker for eating problems and affective disorders among women. J Clin Psychiatry 1988; 49:267–270

311. Mitchell JE, Pomeroy C, Seppala, et al: Pseudo-Bartter's Syndrome, diuretics abuse, idiopathic edema, and eating disorders. Int J Eating Disord 1988; 7:225–237

312. Mitchell JE, Pyle RL, Eckert ED: Frequency and duration of binge-eating episodes in patients with bulimia. Am J Psychiatry 1981; 138:835–836

313. Mitchell JE, Pyle RL, Eckert ED, et al: Electrolyte and other physiological abnormalities in patients with bulimia. Psychol Med 1983; 13:273–278

314. Mitchell, JE, Pyle RL, Eckert ED, et al: Preliminary results of a comparison treatment trial of bulimia nervosa, in The Psychobiology of Bulimia. Edited by Pirke KM, Vandereycken W, Ploog D. Berlin: Springer-Verlag, 1988

315. Mitchell JE, Pyle R, Hatsukami D, et al: Chewing and spitting out food as a clinical feature of bulimia. Psychosomatics 1988; 29:81–84

316. Mitchell JE, Pyle RL, Hatsukami D, et al: The dexamethasone suppression test in patients with bulimia. J Clin Psychiatry 1984; 45:508–511

317. Mitchell JE, Pyle RL, Miner RA: Gastric dilatation as a complication of bulimia. Psychosomatics 1982; 23:96-97

318. Mitchell JE, Seim HC, Colon E, et al: Medical complications and medical management of bulimia. Ann Intern Med 1987:107:71-77

319. Mofenson HC, Caraccio TR: Benefits/risks of syrup of ipecac. Pediatrics 1986; 77:551-552

320. Moldawsky RJ: Myopathy and ipecac abuse in a bulimic patient. Psychosomatics 1985; 26:448-449

321. Morley JE, Bartness TJ, Gosnell BA, et al: Peptidergic regulation of feeding. Int Rev Neurobiol 1985; 27:207-298

322. Morley JE, Blundell JE: The neurobiological basis of eating disorder: Some Formulations. Biol Psychyiatry 1988; 23:53-78

323. Morley JE, Levine AS: The pharmacology of eating behavior. Ann Rev Pharmacol Toxicol 1985; 25:127-46

324. Morley JE, Levine AS: Stress induced eating is mediated through endogenous opiates. Science 1980; 209:1259-1261

325. Morley JE, Levine AS, Gosnell BA, et al: Peptides and feeding. Peptides 1985; 6:181-192

326. Moss RA, Jenning G, McFarland JH, et al: Binge-eating, vomiting and weight fear in a female high school population. J Fam Prac 1984; 18:313-320

327. Musisi S, Garfinkel P: Comparative dexamethasone suppression test measurements in bulimia, depression and normal controls. Can Psychiatr Assoc J 1985; 30:190-194

328. Negus TW, Todd JO: Bulimia nervosa in a male. Br Dent J 1986; 160:290-291

329. Nevo S: Bulimic symptoms: Prevalence and ethnic differences among college women. Int J Eat Dis 1985; 4:151-168

330. Newman MM, Halmi KA: The endocrinology of anorexia nervosa and bulimia nervosa. Endocrinol Metab Clin North Am 1988; 17:195-212

331. Niiya K, Kitagawa T, Fujishita M, et al: Bulimia nervosa complicated by deficiency of vitamin K-dependent coagulation factors. JAMA 1983; 250:792-793

332. Noble RE: Effect of cyproheptadine on appetite and weight gain in adults. JAMA 1969; 209:2054-2055

333. Noble RE: Phenylpropanolamine and blood pressure. The Lancet 1982; 1419

334. Nogami Y, Yabana F: On kabarashi-gui (binge-eating). Folia Psychiatr Neurol Jpn 1977; 31:159-166

335. Norman DK, Herzog DB: A three year outcome study in normal weight bulimia: Assessment of psychosocial functioning and eating attitudes. Psychiatr Res 1986; 19:199-205

336. Norman DK, Herzog DB: Persistent social maladjustment in bulimia: A 1-year follow-up. Am J Psychiatry 1984; 141:444-446

337. Norman DK, Herzog DB, Chauncey S: A one-year outcome study of bulima: Psychological and eating symptom changes in a treatment and non-treatment group. Int J Eating Disord 1986; 5:47-57

338. Norris DL: The effects of mirror confrontation on self-estimation of body dimensions in anorexia nervosa, bulimia and two control groups. Psychol Med 1984; 14:835-842

339. Norris PD, O'Malley BP, Palmer RL: The TRH test in bulimia and anorexia nervosa: A controlled study. J Psychiat Res 1985; 19:215-219

340. O'Brien G, Hassanyeh F, Leake A: The dexamethasone suppression test in bulimia nervosa. Br J Psychiatry 1988; 152:654-656

341. Ong YL, Checkley SA, Russell GFM: Suppression of bulimic symptoms with methylamphetamine. Brit J Psychiatr 1983; 143:288-293

342. Oppenheimer R, Howells K, Palmer RL, et al: Adverse sexual experience in childhood and clinical eating disorders: A preliminary description. J Psychiatr Res 1985; 19:357-361

343. Ordman AM, Kirschenbaum DS: Bulimia: Assessment of eating psychological adjustment, and familial characteristics. Int J Eating Disord 1986; 5:865–878

344. Ordman AM, Kirschenbaum DS: Cognitive behavioral therapy for bulimia: An initial outcome study. J Consult Clin Psychol 1985; 53:305–313

345. Owen WP, Halmi KA, Gibbs J, et al: Satiety responses in eating disorders. J Psychiatr Res 1985; 19:279–284

346. Palmer EP, Guay At: Reversible myopathy secondary to abuse of ipecac in patients with major eating disorders. N Engl J Med 1986; 313:1457–1459

347. Perez EL, Blouin J, Blouin A: The dexamethasone suppression test in bulimia: Nonsuppression associated with depression and suboptimal weight. J Clin Psychiatry 1988; 49:94–96

348. Phillips LG, Cunningham J: Esophageal perforation. Radiol Clin North Am 1984; 22:607–613

349. Piran N, Kennedy S, Garfinkel PE, et al: Eating disorders, affective illness, and borderline personality disorder. J Clin Psychiatry 1988; 49:125

350. Pirke KM, Fichter MM, Chlond C, et al: Disturbances of the menstrual cycle in bulimia nervosa. Clin Endocrinol 1987; 27:245–251

351. Pirke KM, Fichter MM, Schweiger U, et al: Gonadotropin secretion pattern in bulimia nervosa. Int J Eating Disord 1987; 6:655–661

352. Pirke KM, Pahl J, Schweiger U: Metabolic and endocrine indices of starvation in bulimia: A comparison with anorexia nervosa. Psychiatr Res 1985; 14:13–39

353. Pirke KM, Riedel W, Tuschl R, et al: Effect of standardized test meals on plasma norepinephrine in patients with anorexia nervosa and bulima. Int J Eating Disord 1988; 7:369–373

354. Pirke KM, Schweiger U, Laessle R: Metabolic and endocrine consequences of eating behavior and food composition in bulimia. The Psychobiology of Bulimia. Edited by Hudson JI, Pope HG. Washington, DC: American Psychiatric Press, Inc., 1987

355. Pi-Sunyer X, Kissileff HR, Thornton J, et al: C-Terminal octapeptide of cholecystokinin decreases food intake in obese men. Physiol Behav 1983; 29:627–630

356. Polivy J, Herman CP: Dieting and Binging: A causal analysis. Am Psychol 1985; 40:193–201

357. Pope HG, Champoux RF, Hudson JI: Eating disorder and socioeconomic class: Anorexia nervosa and bulimia in nine communities. J Nerv Ment Dis 1987; 175:620–623

358. Pope HG, Frankenburg FR, Hudson JI, et al: Is bulimia associated with borderline personality disorder? A controlled study. J Clin Psychiatry 1987; 48:181–184

359. Pope HG, Hudson JI: Antidepressant drug therapy for bulimia: Current status. J Clin Psychiatry 1986; 47:339–345

360. Pope HG, Hudson JI: Treatment of bulimia with antidepressants. Psychopharmacology 1982; 78:176–179

361. Pope HG, Hudson JI, Jonas JM, et al: Antidepressant treatment of bulimia: A two-year follow-up study. J Clin Psychopharmacol 1985; 5:320–327

362. Pope HG, Jr, Hudson JI, Jonas JM, et al: Bulimia treated with imipramine: A placebo-controlled, double-blind study. Am J Psychiatry 1983; 140:554–558.

363. Pope HG, Hudson JI, Nixon RA, et al: The epidemiology of ipecac abuse. N Engl J Med 1986; 314:245

364. Pope HG, Hudson JI; Yurgelun-Todd D: Anorexia nervosa and bulimia among 300 suburban women shoppers. Am J Psychiatry 1984; 141:292–294

365. Pope HG, Jr, Hudson JI, Yurgelun-Todd D, et al: Prevalence of anorexia nervosa and bulimia in three student populations. Int J Eating Disord 1984; 3:45–51

366. Powers PS, Schulman RG, Gleghorn AA, et al: Perceptual and cognitive abnormalities in bulimia. Am J Psychiatry 1987; 144:1456–1460

367. Powers PS, Fernandez RC: Current treatment of anorexia nervosa and bulimia. Basel, Switzerland: S. Karger AG, 1984

368. Pyle RL: The epidemiology of eating disorders. Pediatrician 1985; 12:102–109

369. Pyle RL, Halvorson PA, Neuman PA, et al: The increasing prevalence of bulimia in freshman college students. Int J Eating Disord 1986; 5:631–647

370. Pyle RL, Mitchell JE: The prevalence of bulimia in selected samples. Ann Am Soc Adolescent Psychiat 1986; 13:241–252

371. Pyle RL, Mitchell JE, Eckert ED: Bulimia: A report of 34 cases. J Clin Psychiatry 1981; 42:60–64

372. Pyle RL, Mitchell JE, Eckert ED: The use of weight tables to categorize patients with eating disorders. Int J Eating Disord 1986; 5:377–383

373. Pyle RL, Mitchell JE Eckert ED, et al: The incidence of bulimia in freshman college students. Int J Eating Disord 1983; 2:75–85

374. Rau JH, Green RS: Compulsive eating: A neuropsychological approach to certain eating disorders. Compr Psychiatry 1975; 16:223–231

375. Rau JH, Green RS: Soft neurological correlates of compulsive eaters. J Nerv Ment Dis 1978; 166:435–437

376. Rau JH, Struve FA, Green RS: Electroencephalographic correlates of compulsive eating. Clin Electroencephalogr 1979; 10:180–189

377. Rauch SD, Herzog DB: Parotidectomy for bulimia: A dissenting view. Am J Otolaryngol 1987; 8:376–380

378. Remick RA, Jones MW, Campos PE: Postictal bulimia. J Clin Psychiatry 1980; 41:256

379. Riemann JF, Schmidt H: Ultrastructural changes in the gut autonomic nervous system following laxative abuse and in other conditions. Scand J Gastroenterology 1982; 71:111–124

380. Robinson P, Grossi L: Gag reflex in bulimia nervosa. Lancet II:221, 1986

381. Robinson PH, Checkley SA, Russell GFM: Suppression of eating by fenfluramine in patients with bulimia nervosa. Br J Psychiatry 1985; 146:169–176

382. Robinson PH, Clarke M, Barrett J: Determinants of delayed gastric emptying in anorexia nervosa and bulimia nervosa. Br Med J 1986; 29:458–464

383. Robinson PH, Holden NL: Bulimia nervosa in the male: A report of nine cases. Psychol Med 1986; 16:795–803

384. Rodman JS, Reidenberg MM: Symptomatic hypokalemia resulting from surreptitious diuretic ingestion. JAMA 1981; 246:1687–1689

385. Rosen JC, Leitenberg H: Bulimia nervosa: Treatment with exposure and response prevention. Behav Ther 1982; 13:117–124

386. Rosen JC, Leitenberg H: Exposure plus response prevention treatment of bulimia nervosa. In Garner DM, Garfinkel PE (Eds), A Handbook of Psychotherapy for Anorexia Nervosa and Bulimia. New York: Guilford Press, 1985

387. Rosen JC, Leitenberg H, Fisher C, et al: Binge-eating episodes in bulimia nervosa: The amount and type of food consumed. Int J Eating Disord 1986; 5:255–267

388. Rosenblum M, Simpson DP, Evenson M: Factitious Bartter's syndrome. Arch Intern Med 1977; 137:1244–1245

389. Rosmark B, Berne C, Holmgren S, et al: Eating disorders in patients with insulin-dependent diabetes mellitus. J Clin Psychiatry 1986; 47:547–550

390. Russell G: Bulimia nervosa: an ominous variant of anorexia nervosa. Psychol Med 1979; 9:429–488

391. Russell GFM: Anorexia nervosa and bulimia nervosa. In Russell GFM, Hersov LA (Eds), Handbook of Psychiatry: The neuroses and personality disorders. New York: Cambridge University Press, 1983

392. Sabine EJ, Yonace A, Farrington AJ, et al: Bulimia nervosa: A placebo-controlled, double-blind therapeutic trial of mianserin. Br J Clin Pharmacol 1983; 15:195S–202S.

393. Saltzman MB: Phenylpropanolamine. Am Fam Physician 1983; 27:23–26.

394. Sato A, Hino N: A case suspected of pseudo-Bartter syndrome. Iryo 1978; 32:1121–1125

395. Saul SH, Dekker A, Watson CG: Acute gastric dilatation with infarction and perforation. Gut 1981; 22:978–983

396. Schneider JA, Agras WS: Bulimia in males: A matched comparison with females. Int J Eating Disord 1987; 235–242

397. Schneider JA, O'Leary A, Agras WS: The role of perceived self-efficacy in recovery from bulimia: A preliminary examination. Behav Res Ther, 1987; 25:429–432

398. Schotte DE, Stunkard AJ: Bulimia vs bulimic behaviors on a college campus. JAMA 1987; 258:1213–1215

399. Schumaker JF, Groth-Marnat G, Small L, et al: Sensation seeking in a female bulimic population. Psychol Rep 1986; 59:1151–1154

400. Schuster CJ, Weil MH, Besso J, et al: Blood volume following diuresis induced by furosemide. Am J Med 1984; 76:585

401. Schwartz BK, Clendinning WE: A cutaneous sign of bulimia. J Am Acad Dermatol 1985; 12:725–726

402. Schwartz DM, Thompson MG, Johnson CL: Anorexia nervosa and bulimia: The sociocultural context. Int J Eating Disord 1:20–36

403. Schwartz HJ: Bulimia: Psychoanalytic perspectives. J Am Psychoanal Assoc 1986; 34:439–62

404. Shapiro SR: Hypertension due to anorectic agent. N Engl J Med 1977; 280:1363

405. Shaw MJ, Hughes JJ, Morley JE: Cholecystokinin octapeptide action on gastric emptying and food intake in normal and vagotomized man. Ann NY Acad Sci 1985; 448, 640–641

406. Shefer T: 'Abnormal' eating attitudes and behaviours among women students. S Afr Med J 1987; 72:419–421

407. Short DD, Blinder BB: Nicotine used as an emetic by a patient with bulimia. Letter to the editor of Am J Psychiatry 1985; 142:272

408. Sights JR, Richards H: Parents of bulimic women. Int J Eating Disord 1984; 3:3–13

409. Silber W: The spectrum of emetogenic injury to the oesophagus. S Afr J Surg 1978; 16:111–119

410. Silva OL: The not-so-harmless laxative. Arch Intern Med 1978; 138:1067

411. Silverstone T, Schuyler D: The effect of cyproheptadine on hunger, caloric intake and body weight in man. Psychopharmacol 1975; 40:335–340

412. Simmons KM: Possible new relief for premenstrual syndrome. JAMA 1983; 250:1371

413. Simmons MS, Grayden SK, Mitchell JE: Bulimia: The need for psychiatric-dental liaison. Am J Psychiatry 1986; 143:783–784

414. Simon D, Laudenbach P, Lebovici M, et al: Parotidomegalie au cours des dysorexies mentales. Nouv Presse Med 1979; 8:2399–2402

415. Simpson MA: Female gential self-mutilation. Arch Gen Psychiatry 1973; 29:808–810

416. Smith GP: The peripheral control of appetite. Lancet 1983; 2:88–89

417. Stacher G, Steinringer H, Schmierer G: Cholecystokinin octapeptide decreases intake of solid food in man. Peptides 1982; 1:133–136

418. Stangler RS, Printz AM: DSM-III: Psychiatric diagnosis in a university population. Am J Psychiatry 1980; 137:937–940

419. Steinmetz PR, Koepper BM: Cellular mechanisms of diuretic action along the nephron. Hosp Prac 1984; 19:125–134

420. Stern SL, Dixon KN, Nemzer E, et al: Affective disorder in the families of women with normal weight bulimia. Am J Psychiatry 1984; 141:1224–1227

421. Sternbach HA, Annitto W, Pottash ALC, et al: Anorexic effects of naltrexone in man. Lancet 1982; I:388–389

422. Striegel-Moore RH, Silberstein LR, Rodin J: Toward an understanding of risk factors for bulimia. Am Psychol 1986; 41:246–263

423. Strober M: The significance of bulimia in juvenile anorexia nervosa: An exploration of possible etiologic factors. Int J Eating Disord 1981; 1:28–43

424. Strober M, Katz J: Depression in the eating disorders: A review and analysis of descriptive, family and biological findings, in Diagnostic Issues in Anorexia Nervosa and Bulimia Nervosa. Garner DM, Garfinkel PE (eds.) New York: Bruner/Mazel, 1988

425. Strober M, Salkin B, Burroughs L, et al: Validity of the bulimia-restrictor distinction in anorexia nervosa: parental personality characteristics and family psychiatric morbidity. J Nerv Ment Dis 1932; 170:345–351

426. Struve FA: Clinical EEG Correlates of Anorexa and Bulimia: Historical review and current findings. Psychiatric Med 1987; 17:927–932

427. Sturdevant RAL, Goetz H: Cholecystokinin both stimulates and inhibits human food intake. Nature 1976; 261:713–715

428. Swartz J: Bulimia: The obsession to be thin. Can Med Assoc J 1984; 130:923–924

429. Swenson RD, Golper TA, Bennett WM: Acute renal failure and rhabdomyolysis after ingestion of phenylpropanolamine-containing diet pills. JAMA 1982; 248:1216

430. Swift TR: Weakness from magnesium-containing cathartics: Electro-physiologic studies. Muscle Nerv 1979; 2:295–298

431. Swift WJ: Assessment of the bulimic patient. Amer J Orthopsychiat 1985; 55:384–396

432. Swift WJ, Andrews D, Barklage NE: The relationship between affective disorder and eating disorders: A review of the literature. Am J Psychiatry 1986; 143:290–299

433. Swift WJ, Kalin NH, Wamboldt FS, et al: Depression in bulimia at 2 to 5 year follow-up. Psychiatr Res 1985; 16:111–122

434. Swift WJ, Ritholz M, Kalin NH, et al: A follow-up study of thirty hospitalized bulimics. Psychosom Med 1987; 49:45–55

435. Szmukler GI: Anorexia nervosa and bulimia in diabetics. J Psychosom Res 1984; 28:365–369

436. Tajiri J, Nakayama M, Sato T, et al: Pseudo-Bartter's syndrome due to furosemide abuse: Report of a case and an analytic review of the Japanese literature. Jpn J Med 1981; 20:216–221

437. Takeuchi T, Koizumi J, Kotsuki H, et al: A clinical study of 30 wrist cutters. Jpn J Psychiatry Neurol 1986; 40:571–581

438. Tamai H, Karibe C, Kiyohara K, et al: Abnormal serum prolactin responses to luteinizing hormone-releasing hormone (LHRH) in patients with anorexia nervosa and bulimia. Psychoneuroendocrinology 1987; 12:281–287

439. Taylor VE, Sneddon J: Bilateral facial swelling in bulimia. Br Dent J 1987; 163:115–117

440. Thelen MH, Mann LM, Pruitt J, et al: Bulimia: Prevalence and component factors in college women. J Psychsom Res 1987; 31:73–78

441. Toner BB, Garfinkel PE, Garner DM: Cognitive style of patients with bulimic and diet-restricting anorexia nervosa. Am J Psychiatry 1987; 144:510–512

442. Touyz SW, Beumont, PJV, Collins, et al: Body shape perception in bulimia and anorexia nervosa. Int J Eating Disord 1985; 4:259–265

443. Touyz SW, Ivison DJ: The prevalence of bulimia in an Australian university sample, in Eating Disorders: Prevalence and Treatment. Edited by Touyz SW, Beumont PJV. Sydney: Williams and Wilkins/Adis, 1985; pp 52–61

444. Turnbull J, Barry F, Annandale A: Physical and Psychological characteristics of five male bulimics. Br J Psychiatry 1987; 150:25–29

445. Ullrich I, Lizarralde G: Amenorrhea and edema. Am J Med 1978; 64:1080–1083

446. Van den Broucke S, Vandereycken W: Anorexia and bulimia nervosa in married patients: A review. Compr Psychiatry 1988; 29:165–173

447. Vandereycken W: Are anorexia nervosa and bulimia variants of affective disorders? Acta Psychiatr Belg 1987; 87:267–280

448. Vandereycken W: Organization and evaluation of an inpatient treatment program for eating disorders. Behav Residential Treat 1988; 3:153–165

449. Vandereychen W: The constructive family approach to eating disorders: Critical remarks on the use of family therapy in anorexia nervosa and bulimia. Int J Eating Disord 1987; 6:455–467

450. VanThorre MD, Vogel FX: The presence of bulimia in high school females. Adolescence 1985; 20:45–51

451. Veale DMW: Exercise dependence. Br J Addict 1987; 82:735–740

452. Viesselman JO, Roig M: Depression and suicidality in eating disorders. J Clin Psychiatry 1985; 46:118–124

453. Vigersky RA, Loriaux DL: The effect of cyproheptadine in anorexia nervosa: A double-blind trial, in Anorexia Nervosa. Edited by Vigersky RA. New York, Raven Press, 1977

454. Wagner S, Halmi KA, Maguire TV: The sense of personal ineffectiveness in patients with eating disorders: One construct or several. Int J Eating Disord 1987; 6:495–505

455. Waller DA, Kiser RS, Hardy BW: Eating behavior and plasma beta endorphin in bulimia. Am J Clin Nutr 1986; 44:20–23

456. Walsh BT, Gladis M, Roose SP, et al: Phenelzine vs placebo in 50 patients with bulimia. Arch Gen Psychiatry 1988; 45:471–475

457. Walsh BT, Lo ES, Cooper T, et al: Dexamethasone suppression test and plasma dexamethasone levels in bulimia. Arch Gen Psychiatry 1987; 44:797–800

458. Walsh BT, Roose SP, Glassman AH, et al: Bulimia and Depression. Psychosom Med 1985; 47:123–131

459. Walsh BT, Stewart JW, Roose SP, et al: Treatment of bulimia with phenelzine. A double-blind, placebo-controlled study. Arch Gen Psychiatry 1984; 41:1105–1109

460. Walsh BT, Stewart JW, Wright L, et al: Treatment of bulimia with monoamine oxidase inhibitors. Am J Psychiatry 1982; 139:1629–1630

461. Walsh BT, Goetz R, Roose SP, et al: EEG-monitored sleep in anorexia nervosa and bulimia. Biol Psychiatry 1985; 20:947–956

462. Wamboldt FS, Kaslow NJ, Swift WJ, et al: Short-term course of depressive symptoms in patients with eating disorders. Am J Psychiatry 1987; 144:362–364

463. Wardle J, Beinart H: Binge-eating: A theoretical review. Br J Clin Psychol 1981; 20:97–109

464. Weingarten HP, Hendler R, Rodin J: Metabolism and endocrine secretion in response to a test meal in normal-weight bulimic women. Psychosom Med 1988; 50:273–285

465. Weisberg LJ, Norman DK, Herzog DB: Personality functioning in normal weight bulimia. Int J Eating Disord 1987; 6:615–631

466. Weiss SR, Ebert MH: Psychological and behavioral characteristics of normal weight bulimics and normal weight controls. Psychosom Med 1983; 45:293–303

467. Weiss BD, Wood GA: Laxative abuse causing gastrointestinal bleeding. J Fam Prac 1982; 15:177–181

468. Wegner JT, Struve FA: Incidence of the 14 and 6 per second position spike pattern in an adult clinical population: An empirical note. J Nerv Ment Dis 1977; 164:340–345

469. Weilberg JB, Stakes JW, Brotman A, et al: Sleep architecture in bulimia: A pilot study. Biol Psychiatry 1985; 30:225–228

470. Wermuth BM, Davis RL, Hollister LE, et al: Phenytoin treatment of binge-eating syndrome. Am J Psychiatry 1977; 134:1249–1253

471. White WC, Boskind-White M: An experiential-behavioral approach to the treatment of

bulimarexia. Psychotherapy: Theory, Research and Practice, vol. 18, no. 4, Winter 1981, pp. 501–507

472. Williamson DA, Kelley ML, Davis CJ, et al: Psychopathology of eating disorders: A controlled comparison of bulimic, obese, and normal subjects. J Consult Clin Psychol 1985; 53:161–166

473. Wilson CP (Ed): Fear of Being Fat: The Treatment of Anorexia Nervosa and Bulimia. New York: Jason Aronson, 1983

474. Wilson GT, Lindholm L: Bulimia nervosa and depression. Int J Eat Dis 1987; 6:725–732

475. Wilson GT, Rossiter E, Kleifield EI, et al: Cognitive behavioral treatment of bulimia nervosa: A controlled evaluation. Behav Res Ther 1986; 24:277–288

476. Wilson T: Assessing treatment outcome in bulimia nervosa: A methodological note. Int J Eating Disord 1987; 6:339–348

477. Winstead DK, Willard SG: Bulimia: Diagnostic clues. South Med J 1983; 76:313–315

478. Wolchik SA, Weiss L, Katzman MA: An empirically validated, short-term psychoeducational group treatment program for bulimia. Int J Eating Disord 1986; 5:21–34

479. Wolcott RB, Yager J, Gordon G: Dental sequelae to the binge-purge syndrome (bulimia): Report of cases. JAMA 1984; 109:723–725

480. Wold PN: Family attitudes toward weight in bulimia and in affective disorder–A pilot study. Psychiatr J of Univ of Ottawa 1985; 10:162–164

481. Wurtman JJ: Carbohydrate craving: A disorder of food intake and mood, in The Psychobiology of Bulimia. Edited by Hudson JI, Pope HG. Washington, DC: American Psychiatric Press, Inc., 1987; pp 231–239

482. Wurtman J, Wurtman R, Mark S, et al: d-fenfluramine selectively suppresses carbohydrate snacking by obese subjects. Int J Eating Disord 1985; 4:89–99

483. Wynn DR, Martin MJ: A physical sign of bulimia (Letter). Mayo Clin Proc 1984; 59:722

484. Yager J, Landsverk J, Edelstein CK: A 20-month follow-up study of 628 women with eating disorders, I: Course and Severity. Am J Psychiatry 1987; 144:1172–1177

485. Yates AJ, Sambrailo F: Bulimia nervosa: A descriptive and therapeutic study. Behav Res Ther 1984; 22:503–517

486. Zinkand H, Cadoret RJ, Widmer RB: Incidence and detection of bulimia in a family practice population. J Fam Pract 1984; 18:555–560

487. Zuckerman DM, Colby A, Ware NC, et al: The prevalence of bulimia among college students. Am J Public Health 1986; 76:1135–1137

Index

Index

AA (Alcoholics Anomymous) 98

Abnormal GH responses to TRH in bulimia (table 16), 64

Abstinence: abrupt vs. gradual interruption of target behaviors, 97–98, 100; pure abstinence model, 98; pure CBT model, 98; rapid interruption model, 99

"Abstinence," pros and cons of, 98

Acidosis, 43

Affective disorder, 3, 61, 80, 89, 101, 104; diagnosis in patients with bulimia nervosa (table 7), 25; and obese bulimics, 9

Age of onset of bulimia nervosa, 9

Alcohol/drug abuse, 3, 27–29

Alkalosis, 43

Anorexia nervosa, 38, 40, 55, 61; DSM-III-R diagnosis of, 8; subgroups described, 100

Anticonvulsants, 85

Antidepressant drugs, 89, 90; amitriptyline, 81; bupropion, 82; desipramine, 82; imipramine, 81, 82, 84; length of drug therapy, 93; MAO (monoamine oxidase inhibitors), 81, 84; mianserin, 81; overview of available heterocyclics (table 19), 90; side effects/adverse reactions— tricyclics (table 20), 92

Antidepressant treatment: involvement, completion, and outcomes (table 18), 83; overview of studies in bulimia nervosa (table 17), 82

Anxiety, 56

APA (American Psychiatric Association): bulimia nervosa formally recognized by, 6

Behavioral disorder, 4

Behavioral chain illustrating typical bulimic pattern (figure 8), 137

Bemis, K. M., 98, 120

Beta hydroxybutyric acid, 62

Binge-eating, 6, 7, 13, 16–18, 28, 107; definition of, 16; in DSM-III-R criteria, 7–8; duration of, 17; macronutrient content of, 18; prevalence of, 13, 16–17

Body image disturbance, 29; counseling of, 138–40; treatment of, 138–40

Body inventory (table 28), 139

Borderline personality disorder and bulimia (table 27), 27

Boskind-Lodahl, M., and White, W. C., 105

Brewerton, T. D., 58

Bruch, H., 120

Bulik, C. M., 28

Bulimia nervosa: age of onset, 9; and alcohol/drug abuse, 3, 27–29, 103; and antidepressants, 26, 55, 57, 88, 89; as a behavioral disorder, 4; and borderline personality disorder (table 8), 27; characteristics of (table 4), 10; in college-age women, 11; defined, 3–4; demography of, 9–11; and depression, 3–4, 11, 24–26, 102; diagnostic criteria, 13; diagnostic systems of, 6; duration of, 11; epidemiology of, 11, 13; and family problems, 30; follow-up studies (table 6) of, 14; and gender, 5, 9; in general population, 11; and impulsivity, 30; in industrialized societies, 5; longitudinal course of, 14; and low self-esteem, 4,

James E. Mitchell, M.D., is associate professor of psychiatry at the University of Minnesota, where he has been a faculty member since 1979. He earned his M.D. degree from Northwestern University Medical School and served his internship in internal medicine at the Indiana University Hospitals and his residency in psychiatry at the University of Minnesota. He has been active in teaching, clinical work, and research in the area of eating disorders since that time. Among his many activities, he serves on the editorial board of the *International Journal of Eating Disorders*, the International Advisory Committee of the Anorexic Aid Society, and the American Psychiatric Association Task Force on DSM-IV Eating Disorders Committee. He edited the book *Anorexia Nervosa and Bulimia: Diagnosis and Treatment* (Minnesota 1985) and contributes regularly to scientific journals, including the *International Journal of Eating Disorders*, the *American Journal of Psychiatry*, and *Biological Psychiatry*.